Understanding Research in
Complementary and Alternative Medicine

A guide to reading and analysing research in healthcare

Edzard Ernst MD PhD FRCP FRCPEd

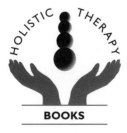

HOLISTIC THERAPY

BOOKS

Published by Holistic Therapy Books

An imprint of Ruben Publishing, part of Education and Media Services Ltd.

8 Station Court, Station Road, Great Shelford,

Cambridge, CB22 5NE

Tel: 0870 242 7867

Fax: 01223 846445

© Education & Media Services Ltd 2007.

First published October 2007

ISBN 978-1-903348-09-3

Set in 8/12 Foundry Form Sans Book

Printed by Scotprint, Haddington

Prepared for the publishers by The Write Idea, Cambridge

CONTENTS

PREFACE

Separating fact from fiction

I have often thought it regrettable how little knowledge and understanding some healthcare practitioners (HCPs) have in research. With that term, HCP, I am here including practitioners of complementary and alternative medicine (CAM), nurses, physiotherapists, radiotherapists and others – all professionals working with patients and clients day in, day out, who have not studied formal medicine and have therefore had little or no exposure to research methodology teaching.

The term is awkward, I admit, but I like "professions allied to medicine" or other options even less. The lack of interest in research, I suspect, is at least partly due to a lack of an understanding about what research is about. Research is a way of finding the truth and separating it from opinion. Of course, science does not have all the answers but it delivers the facts. In turn the facts enable us to make the right decisions.

True, research is not always an easy subject, but once you put your mind to it you will be surprised how straight forward it usually is. Anyone can grasp its basic principles, and anyone working with patients should. You don't need to be a "mastermind" to understand the concept of testing treatments for efficacy and safety or to comprehend the idea of evidence-based medicine.

Through reading this book as you prepare for, or during, your professional life, you will be able to understand the essential concepts of medical and healthcare research. This, in turn, will enable you to work in your profession understanding and using the ideas and developments that you learn from reading research so that you can incorporate them into your practice. If enough therapists do this it is a step towards improving the healthcare of the future. It could well become a major part of your own Continuous Professional Development.

Structure of this book

This book was written to be used in two different ways. The central section 'Important concepts and explanations' is an A–Z guide. You can use it to look up terms that you come across when reading research papers, and you can employ it to obtain explanations for key terms used in the rest of the text. These are highlighted **like this**. It will enable you to reference these terms and quickly find out what each means.

Prior to and after this central section, the book is set out to give you an explanation of how research works with examples for you to become able to read research articles and paper. This provides an introduction to research methodology, which will be invaluable to those new to their professions and new to the need to understand research reports.

In whichever way you use the book, I hope you find it valuable. After reading it you may have to give up a prejudice treasured by many for a long time: medical research is not boring, inaccessible or irrelevant at all. It is the best method we have for separating fact from fiction.

Edzard Ernst

Feedback

The author and publisher are interested in comments by readers to inform future editions. Please send any comments to sales@holistic-books.co.uk.

CHAPTER 1 WHY RESEARCH?

And if the blind lead the blind, both shall fall into the ditch (Matthew 15:14)

Recently the 'British Medical Journal' conducted a survey to determine the greatest medical discoveries since the journal was first published in 1840. About one hundred important breakthroughs were nominated. A panel then narrowed them down to 15:

- Anaesthesia
- Antibiotics
- Chlorpromazine
- Computers
- Discovery of DNA structure
- Evidence-based medicine
- Germ theory
- Imaging techniques
- Immunology
- Oral rehydration therapy
- The Pill
- Risk of smoking
- Sanitation
- Tissue culture
- Vaccines

What a list! It reminds us how brisk scientific progress has been in just 150 years. Collectively these discoveries have saved billions of lives. Without research, medicine would be impotent. The long history of medicine sadly provides ample proof for that statement.

Distrust of research

Many healthcare practitioners are still not convinced. Some are even deeply distrustful of research. Others are afraid to do it because the results of the research might not show what they hope.

Research, they fear, might therefore be detrimental to their field in general and to their own livelihood in particular. Others again may feel that research is only for the satisfaction of researchers. To me this sounds like claiming bread is good only for bakers. Researchers generate findings which are for healthcare practitioners to implement – to the benefit of the patient.

The importance of finding the truth

Even if the findings really should turn out to be negative in one particular area, this surely would require serious consideration. Either such results are true; then honesty and professional ethics demand that we take them seriously, or they are false; then we should do the research properly so that the truth can be demonstrated.

In any case, it seems essential to understand what research is all about. Without some basic knowledge, healthcare practitioners will remain passive bystanders in a process which is vital to their own futures.

Sadly, we are not born with the ability to understand research – we have to learn the essentials about it. Once we do this, we are likely to find that research can be quite fascinating and, after all, not that difficult either.

In this book, I will explain medical and healthcare research in a way that is understandable for healthcare practitioners. Even if you don't accept that research is necessary, nobody can deny that healthcare practitioners will in future have to comprehend its basic concepts. As many more healthcare practitioners are becoming regulated and progressively integrated into clinical routines, practitioners will have to read and understand the latest research papers. To be fully informed is an ethical imperative for all healthcare providers. This means, *not* being informed is unethical!

'Evidence based' treatments

Increasingly within national health services world wide only treatments that are shown by evidence – not just long use – are being approved. That evidence is provided by proper research being conducted professionally.

CAM treatments are increasingly being requested by the public, but before they can become part of the mainstream of healthcare the claims made need to be fully tested.

Many of the public who use CAM treatments do so alongside conventional medicine

Arguments often used against research and counter-arguments.

I know it works because I see the benefit in my patients/ clients.	OK, but you still need to convince the sceptics, healthcare providers and insurance companies as they increasingly insist on scientific evidence. Perceived effects may be quite unrelated to the therapy in question. It can be caused by a range of factors such as natural history of the disease, placebo-effects, your therapeutic relationship etc.
Clinical trials are not a good method for evaluating my therapy.	Clinical trials are routinely adapted in many ways so that they adequately accommodate any therapy. The fact that many clinical trials of most interventions already exist (and many show positive results) proves that clinical trials are feasible.
My therapy must be individualised which is not possible in clinical trial.	Many clinical trials of individualised treatments already exist – so it is possible.
My therapy is holistic, research just attempts to simplify (be reductionist). The two principles do not go together.	The design of a trial can be adapted such that the holistic nature of your therapy is fully respected.
The effects of my therapy are so subtle that they cannot be measured.	Researchers have developed many extremely subtle outcome measures which capture, for instance, quality of life, well-being or patient preference.
I have no time to learn all this difficult stuff.	First it is not difficult and second this 'stuff' is important. You should take the time.

often without telling their medical practitioners. They do this because they fear the reaction of their doctors who feel may be biased against these 'alternative' methods. Without a evidence base it is likely that this bias will continue.

A great deal of research has already been undertaken and needs to be read and understood by healthcare practitioners. Also new research needs to be undertaken. (See Chapter 7 for a full discussion on evidence-based medicine.)

The value of this book

What I hope you will achieve with this book can be summarised as follows:

- You should obtain sufficient background knowledge to be able to comprehend the details of a published research paper. This includes the identification of its strengths and weaknesses – so that you are in a position, for instance, to criticise its conclusion, if necessary.
- Once you understand 'the basics', you should be able to further develop your own research interests. This could mean getting involved in research projects yourself or participating in discussions and debates about the evidence for or against a given therapeutic approach. Secretly, I hope you will be 'infected' by the passion I feel for research.
- Eventually this might contribute to a 'culture change'. By this I mean a situation where healthcare professionals are no longer outsiders to research in their own area but are active, well-informed partners in it.

Ultimately, my vision is for all of us to help the best we can improving future healthcare. I know we are aiming high but I think it's worth the effort.

CHAPTER 2 THE RESEARCH PROCESS

What is research?

The object of research is the advancement not of the investigator, but of knowledge. (M. H. Gordon 1872–1953)

Note: Where a word or phrase is in **bold** it is listed alphabetically in the main central section of the book where it is explained in full.

Research is defined as the systematic investigation to establish facts and principles or to collect information on a subject. Systematic means to be methodical, to use order and planning. Thus research can be seen as a tool to find the truth. The hallmark of good research is that it is free of **bias**. Researchers or scientists should not be interested in proving a point, they want to test **hypotheses** or answer **research questions**.

HYPOTHESIS

Hypothesis is used in research and experiments to propose a logical question that is then answered by testing that question to see what in fact the answer is.

The question must be one that can be answered by evidence that can be collected and verifed.

Showing and testing

You might, for instance, read in a paper:
'The aim of this study was to show therapeutic touch is effective for …'.
Whenever you see something like this you should suspect bias. The true aim of the study should be:
'To test whether therapeutic touch is effective for …'.

This may look like a small difference, almost splitting hairs, but the difference is considerable and important. The first is 'to show' which implies that the researcher wanted to prove something he/she already believed; the second is 'to test' which is impartial.

Researchers must be impartial. This obviously is a tall order. Researchers are only human, and as humans we all have preferences, beliefs and interests..

Scientific approach

Being totally objective is therefore an ideal that is hard to reach. Nevertheless, it is essential to make the best effort to approach it and that means minimising **bias**. The way to do this, is to conduct research according to the rules of scientific rigor. This book is all about explaining what this means.

Good or bad methods?

What we call experience is often a dreadful list of ghastly mistakes
(J. Chalmers Da Costa, 1863–1933)

The discussion about what constitutes a good, and what a bad, research method has been going on for many years. It has been particularly lively in complementary and alternative medicine (CAM). Some people, for instance, insist that the concept of the conventional **clinical trial** is ill-suited for the study of therapeutic touch, homeopathy, massage therapy, acupuncture and many other therapies that fall outside the 'medical' area.

For decades, emotional battles were fought between those who favoured a certain research method and those who claimed it was inadequate. In the end, the inescapable conclusion is that most of these debates were based on misunderstandings. They have generated plenty of heat but little light.

The long and short of all this is simple: there is no such thing as a good or bad research method. All research tools are at the same time potentially good and potentially bad. What matters foremost is to apply the right tool for the right task. Nobody would use a spade to tighten a screw or a screwdriver to dig a hole. Similarly, it would be silly to determine the popularity of a treatment with a **randomised clinical trial** . The fact that a spade is of no use for tightening a screw does not mean it is a useless tool itself. The fact that a randomised clinical trial is inadequate for some research questions does not render it useless for other types of investigation.

The right method for the right question

The crucial and rather obvious point is that the tool needs to be matched to the task at hand. For each task, there is a tool which is well-suited and dozens which are not. For each **research question** there is an adequate research method and many which are inadequate. What follows is disarmingly simple: there are no good or bad research methods but only good or bad matches between research questions and research methods.

Types of research methods

It is important to understand the vales of the various types of research methods that are available. Two broad categories exist: qualitative and quantitative.

AN EXAMPLE OF QUALITATIVE RESEARCH

Below is a extract from the summary of an article.

'The burgeoning interest in complementary therapies (CTs) in the general population over the last decade has created a demand for CTs to be made available within the NHS. There are some excellent examples of midwives who have introduced CTs into clinical practice and who are providing an enhanced service to women as a result.

Result
Overall, however, service provision remains patchy and ad hoc with little evidence of a robust integration into the maternity services.

This article presents the qualitative findings from a national survey of the heads of maternity services in England. They were asked to indicate their views and perceptions about the benefits, promoters and constrainers in relation to CT integration within the maternity services. Our findings show that overall, views are positive, with increasing consumer satisfaction, promotion of normal childbirth and a reduction in medical intervention being seen as the main benefits.'

The findings indicate that there is now the opportunity to do research to test out if these no doubt honestly held 'views' can be confirmed through proper analysis.

Julie Williams and Mary Mitchell, Senior Lecturers in Midwifery, University of West of England, Bristol.

(See PubMed – indexed for MEDLINE)

Qualitative research

Qualitative research is about determining people's opinions, beliefs, attitudes, knowledge, behaviours etc. Essentially it is descriptive by nature. It does not test hypotheses or measure outcomes – meaning it does not normally generate numbers and statistics. Its domain is to interpret phenomena, give them meaning and to generate (rather than test) hypotheses.

Typical qualitative research projects could be:
- to generate cancer patients' views on the quality of nursing care,
- to describe patients' explanations of their illness,
- to determine why patients prefer physiotherapy to chiropractic or vice versa,
- to describe the barriers encountered when accessing community nursing, complementary therapies etc.

Some of the main methods used for qualitative research are interview studies and focus groups. As with any quantitative research, qualitative research should be rigorous – meaning it should:

- be based on a clear **research question**,
- use appropriate research methods,
- be reproducible,
- recruit the right subjects in the correct context,
- draw conclusions that are based on the findings of the study alone.

A common problem with qualitative research is that its findings may only apply to the particular circumstances of that one investigation – in other words, they may have little **generalisability**. We may therefore not apply the findings to other situations.

Quantitative research

That is the type of research that involves assessment of data – meaning actual numbers and calculations. There are many types of studies. One way to categorise them is to differentiate between observational and experimental investigations.

- A typical experimental study is the **clinical trial**.
- Typical observational studies are **case-control studies** and **cohort studies**.

Most of this book is focussed on quantitative research, particularly the clinical trial. As to the vexed question whether the effectiveness of CAM should be assessed in a **clinical trial** or in an **observational study**, see page 20.

Research questions

Next we should ask ourselves what types of research questions exist. The options are almost limitless. Typical types may include the following:

- Why do certain patients develop certain symptoms or conditions?
- Why do patients make certain choices?
- What are the risks of a certain treatment?
- What are the merits of one approach versus another?
- What do we know about Treatment X?
- How much do nurses, physiotherapists etc know about Treatment X?
- Is a treatment safe?
- Is it effective?
- Is it value for money?

Of course, these are not fully formulated research questions but the list gives a flavour about the variety that exists.

To emphasise it again: it is crucial to find an optimal match between a research question and a research method which could answer them. Let's have a look at a few examples.

Research questions

1. Which type of therapy do people use who suffer from acute back pain? 2. For what conditions do British patients employ acupuncture?	These might be important issues, for instance, when planning health service provision or when designing training courses. A good research tool for such questions might be a **survey** of a representative sample of back pain patients and UK acupuncturists respectively.
3. What do patients expect when they consult an aromatherapist? 4. Why do some people prefer seeing a professional homeopath to consulting their GP?	Such research questions are probably best tackled using qualitative research methods (see above). One could, for instance, consider in depth interviews or **focus groups**.
5. What is the best herbal treatment for preventing migraine?	This is a complex question which might require more than one research method. One could, for instance, start with qualitative research and ask a panel of expert herbalists about their experience. Subsequently one could consider **clinical trials** to test the most promising approaches. Alternatively one might evaluate the existing data by conducting a **systematic review** to find out whether such studies are already available.
6. Are there any risks associated with spinal manipulation?	Safety issues are obviously vitally important. They can be tackled with a range of methods. A reasonable start, for instance, would be to conduct a **systematic review** of all reports of side effects after spinal manipulation.
7. How often do these side-effects occur?	The above review is likely to generate a multitude of reports. It will, however, not tell us whether these adverse events are frequent or rare. To get information on this crucial point, we need a **prospective study**. Ideally we require a representative sample of therapists who regularly perform spinal manipulation to follow-up and document all such patients and the side-effects they might experience. A study of this nature would inform us what proportion of patients experience this or that problem.

8. Does Treatment X work?

This type of question, I'm sure, is for many decision makers the most important one. Some practitioners may not find it that crucial – they are totally convinced that their therapy is effective.

In rare cases, medical treatments are indeed so dramatically effective that no research is required to establish their efficacy. If we are confronted with a patient who cannot drink or eat, for instance, because he is in a coma, it is obvious to artificially feed him.

If we see a patient whose heart has just stopped, it is clear that we try to resuscitate him provided we have the skills. If a patient has lost a lost of blood, we must give him a transfusion. No trials are needed to establish that such interventions work.

Even certain drug treatments were so dramatically effective when they were first discovered, that no-one ever submitted them to clinical trials testing their effectiveness. Examples include the following[1]:

- Insulin for diabetes
- Ether for anaesthesia
- Chemotherapy for testicular cancer
- Sulphanilimide for puerperal sepis
- Streptomycin for tuberculous meningitis

But much of healthcare, including CAM, physiotherapy and nursing, does not fall into that category. More often than not, therapeutic effects are mild, slow to emerge or uncertain altogether. In other words, we need to investigate in order to be sure – and that means we need clinical trials.

Experience

What about experience? Does long experience of providing therapies count for nothing? Are not certain therapies are 'time-tested'?

Healthcare decision makers or advisors will be unimpressed to hear that a particular treatment has been around for hundreds of years and therefore has 'stood the test of time'. We know that this type of evidence is not reliable – think of bloodletting, for instance. It was used for millennia and clearly generated more harm than good. Or think of HRT which was promoted forcefully for many years, and only after rigorous trials emerged, we learned that it was actually not as harmless as previously thought

That is not to say that experience has no value – it means that it cannot be a substitute for scientific proof that will count as 'evidence'.

Similarly, your own experience with a therapy will hardly be considered convincing 'proof'. Nobody would doubt that many of your patients/clients improve after you administered your treatments. But sceptics will caution you that your impressions might be clouded by a range of factors, e.g.

- Those patients who don't improve and possibly even deteriorate simply don't come back – your experience may therefore not tell the whole story.
- Most conditions get better no matter what we do – if you administer Treatment X and your patient improves; they might have improved even without therapy. Think of a common cold or an episode of acute back pain – both usually disappear regardless of whether or how we treat them.
- Many patients use a range of treatments when they are ill and often don't tell you about them – therefore your patient's improvement might have been caused by another therapy.
- If you are kind to someone, as I'm sure you are, they will also be kind to you – this can result in your patient saying they are better only to not disappoint you.
- Every treatment also has a powerful placebo-effect – which means your patient's improvement might not be related to a specific effect of Treatment X but could be due to a **placebo-response**. (Placebo is explained in full in Chapter 7).
- Of course, there is nothing wrong with that – the main thing is that your patient gets better – but theoretically your treatment *could* be a pure placebo. All treatments, even those which are effective beyond placebo, generate a placebo-response. Therefore any therapy that relies solely on the placebo-effect is not optimal. It delivers only part of what your patient deserves.

> **PLACEBO**
>
> This much used term is often misunderstood and even used as a term of abuse. In clinical trials one group may be provided with a treatment which is thought to be wholly inactive but is to the patient/client indistinguishable from the real thing. The results then compare the outcomes of those who had the 'real' treatment to those that had the 'placebo'. Quite often those who have the placebo show improvement as well! **Understanding placebo** is important in all research.

It follows, I think, that we need to make as sure as we possibly can that Treatment X reliably generates specific effects that are clinically useful. The best way to do this is to conduct a clinical trial. However, we need a more precise research question than 'does it work?'

We need to define the treatment, the patient population and what we mean by clinical improvement, i.e. the **outcome measure**. So we might end up with a research question such as this one:

Does Swedish massage reduce the pain of patients suffering from acute back pain?

Of course, this still does not provide all the details – we don't know, for instance, who is administering the treatment, what exactly it entails, how often it is given and for how long. But at least, it provides a basic framework; the details can be provided later.

Controlled clinical trial

One crucial element is, however, still missing. Imagine we carry out the above study by treating 100 patients for 4 weeks. By this time, we can be sure that many of them experience considerably less pain. As explained above, this would also be the case, if they had not received any treatment at all.

There are plenty of other factors which lead to improvement. We therefore need to take them into account. The best way to do this is to conduct a **controlled clinical trial**.

There is nothing complicated about this method. Essentially we treat two groups of patients – one with massage (the '**experimental treatment**') and the other group (the '**control**') in another way. The options for the other way include:

A)   No treatment at all.
B)   A placebo therapy, e.g. sham massage (e.g. slight stoking only).
C)   An active treatment, e.g. the accepted treatment for that condition.

The research question
The optimal choice for the control is determined by your research question. The three options above match up to three different questions:

A)   Is the massage treatment better than doing nothing?
B)   Is it better than placebo?
C)   Is it better than the standard therapy?

These questions are all meaningful in their own right. It is not true to say, this one is good or this one is bad. Your choice will depend on what you want to find out, what you need the results for, or which of the three questions has not yet been conclusively answered by previous research.

Randomised clinical trial

Finally there is a further, rather crucial matter. Imagine that the allocation of patients to the **experimental** or **control group**, in a clinical trial, is influenced by choice. You or the patient might decide which treatment is given. This would inevitably create uneven groups.

In a trial of massage versus no treatment, for instance, those patients choosing massage might differ from those who don't in:

- A)   the severity of their symptoms,
- B)   the medical history,
- C)   sex,
- D)   ethnicity etc.

But the comparison can only work if the two groups are comparable for all factors except for the treatment they receive. If not, who knows, maybe the unevenness influences the result of the study. Any difference in outcome could then be due to that unevenness rather than to the treatment.

False negative result

Imagine, for instance, we end up with a result that implies massage is no better than no treatment at all. The reason could be that the patients in the massage group were worse off to start with – it is likely that, given the choice, those who suffer more pain would elect (or be selected) to receive massage! The results of such a study would therefore suggest massage to be ineffective while, in fact, it is effective. In 'science speak', this would be a '**false negative**' result . It seems clear that such a finding would be grossly misleading. It follows that we need to make one thing quite sure: the groups must be similar, i.e. comparable in all respects.

Randomisation

The best way to achieve this is to allocate patients according to a randomisation code. This sounds complicated but, in fact, it could not be simpler. In essence, randomisation is a process which lets coincidence decide which group each patient is allocated to. Flipping a coin for each patient is perfectly adequate – but there are more elegant, computerised methods as well.

If randomisation is done correctly, its effect is magic: not only are the groups similar in terms of factors known to influence the outcome, e.g. severity of symptom or chronicity of condition. Even factors that are important but currently unknown to us are distributed evenly. Think of genetic predispositions, for instance. The result is that the two groups are entirely comparable.

Observational versus clinical studies

In CAM and other healthcare, many people feel that the clinical trial is not an adequate method – to these people it creates a situation that is artificial and does not reflect 'real life'. Thus they favour observational studies where 'real life' patients 'receive the treatment in 'real life' situations. To comprehend what is really going on, let's choose an example: acupuncture for migraine.

In an observational study, patients would be checked for diagnosis so that we can be sure all suffer from migraine and not some other form of periodic headache. Subsequently they would be asked to monitor the frequency and severity of their symptoms in a diary. Then they would receive regular acupuncture treatments for 4 months. The researchers would then look at all the diaries and calculate average values for migraine frequency and severity.

Let's assume the frequency and severity fell during the 4 months of treatment by 20% and 25% respectively, and both changes are statistically significant, i.e.. not due to chance. Would this prove the effectiveness of acupuncture in treating migraine?

Proponents of observational studies are sure the answer is yes. But sceptics are not convinced. They would point out that a range of factors could have produced this result even in the absence of an effective treatment. These factors include:

1. The placebo-effect – all treatments come with a sizable placebo effect which could, for instance, be due to the patient's expectation of a good result.
2. **'Regression towards the mean'** – patients entering the study are likely to suffer severely at that point, if not they would not have volunteered; as all things oscillate around a mean value, the extreme pain is likely to be less when measured some time later.
3. Concomitant therapies – patients who are suffering are likely to use all sorts of treatments, often without telling their clinicians; thus treatments other than acupuncture could have caused the result.

Therefore sceptics will always insist that the effectiveness is tested in a **controlled clinical trial**. In an ideal world, we need both clinical trials and observational studies. The former tells us whether a treatment *can* work, the latter whether it *will* work in 'real life'.

Anecdotal evidence?

Anecdotal evidence is information obtained from personal accounts, examples and observations. For many clinicians and certainly for most patients this is powerful evidence. Scientists, on the other hand, are usually less impressed. Does that mean that anecdotal evidence is useless?

Value

On the contrary, anecdotal evidence can be of crucial importance. We should, however, bear in mind what is emphasized repeatedly throughout this book: there are no good or bad research methods – only good or bad matches between the research question and the research method.

Forms

Anecdotal evidence can take various forms and shapes. Typically it is the account of one single patient receiving Treatment X for Condition Y. If nothing spectacular happens as a result, we usually don't consider that as important evidence. If the patient does, however, have a remarkable response, it may well amount to something. In the above scenario, the patient might improve or she might experience an adverse event. Both of these reactions can be important.

Positive response

I will consider the positive response first. Let's say our patient has had a serious condition like cancer, she took a natural remedy, and the cancer disappeared. Nobody in his right mind could claim this is not important – after all, we may have stumbled over an effective treatment for a life-threatening condition!

The crux is that we cannot possibly be sure. Perhaps the patient has also been treated with conventional treatments and they caused the cancer to disappear. Perhaps the patient only thought she was suffering from cancer and the diagnosis was never truly established. There is, of course, an important lesson here: anecdotes of this nature need to be recorded meticulously. We need all the information that may be relevant for what effectively then amounts to a proper **case report**.

If detailed information is available, this **case report** would be very valuable indeed. Sadly, however, it would not prove that the remedy administered cured the cancer. Proof would require a proper clinical trial, one single case, even if it is dramatic, can only put us on the right track for further investigation.

Often, anecdotal evidence is far less spectacular. Mostly it relates to cases where things went particularly smoothly or instances where a certain, seemingly minor change in the normal treatment protocol was followed by a particularly positive response. These types of case reports will obviously not change the way we treat cancer but they can inform other practitioners who might learn valuable lessons from them which, in turn, could enhance their future practice.

Adverse response

Perhaps the most important type of case report is the one where a patient suffers an **adverse event**. Just like positive responses, adverse events must be reported in full. All important clinical details should be provided in order to maximise the conclusiveness of the case. But even with the fullest of detail we cannot be sure about cause and effect on the basis of one single such case report.

The situation changes if more and more similar reports are noted. An example is the herbal anxiolytic remedy kava. It is very effective in reducing anxiety and therefore it became hugely popular several years ago. But then, case reports appeared suggesting that it caused liver damage. When about 70 such reports were published worldwide, some national regulators felt they needed to take action and banned the herbal medicine. This story makes it very clear how important case reports or anecdotal evidence can be.

Formulation of hypotheses

Anecdotal evidence can never amount to a scientific proof of anything. What it does, however, is to alert us that something may be going on. Subsequently it is our responsibility to dig deeper and find out what that something is. Put into scientific language: anecdotal evidence cannot test hypotheses but it is well-suited for formulating **hypotheses** which subsequently should be studied in depth with other research tools.

Examples of Good Research

There is plenty of good research. Therefore choosing a few examples is not easy. What follows is a personal selection.

Example 1

On 21st December 2004, six UK national newspapers reported that *'Acupuncture Effectively Relieves Pain of Knee Osteoarthritis'*. The reason for this 'media frenzy' was a study from the US. Here is its abstract available on Medline. Do not be concerned about understanding the statistics at this stage.

BACKGROUND: Evidence on the efficacy of acupuncture for reducing the pain and dysfunction of osteoarthritis is equivocal.

OBJECTIVE: To determine whether acupuncture provides greater pain relief and improved function compared with sham acupuncture or education in patients with osteoarthritis of the knee.

DESIGN: Randomized, controlled trial.

SETTING: Two outpatient clinics (an integrative medicine facility and a rheumatology facility) located in academic teaching hospitals and 1 clinical trials facility.

PATIENTS: 570 patients with osteoarthritis of the knee (mean age [+/-SD], 65.5 +/- 8.4 years).

INTERVENTION: 23 true acupuncture sessions over 26 weeks. Controls received 6 two-hour sessions over 12 weeks or 23 sham acupuncture sessions over 26 weeks.

MEASUREMENTS: Primary outcomes were changes in the Western Ontario and McMaster Universities Osteoarthritis Index (WOMAC) pain and function scores at 8 and 26 weeks. Secondary outcomes were patient global assessment, 6-minute walk distance, and physical health scores of the 36-Item Short-Form Health Survey (SF-36).

RESULTS: Participants in the true acupuncture group experienced greater improvement in WOMAC function scores than the sham acupuncture group at 8 weeks (mean difference, -2.9 [95% CI, -5.0 to -0.8]; $P = 0.01$) but not in WOMAC pain score (mean difference, -0.5 [CI, -1.2 to 0.2]; $P = 0.18$) or the patient global assessment (mean difference, 0.16 [CI, -0.02 to 0.34]; $P > 0.2$). At 26 weeks, the true acupuncture group experienced significantly greater improvement than the sham group in the WOMAC function score (mean difference, -2.5 [CI, -4.7 to -0.4]; $P = 0.01$), WOMAC pain score (mean difference, -0.87 [CI, -1.58 to -0.16]; $P = 0.003$), and patient global assessment (mean difference, 0.26 [CI, 0.07 to 0.45]; $P = 0.02$).

LIMITATIONS: At 26 weeks, 43% of the participants in the education group and 25% in each of the true and sham acupuncture groups were not available for analysis.

CONCLUSIONS: Acupuncture seems to provide improvement in function and pain relief as an adjunctive therapy for osteoarthritis of the knee when compared with credible sham acupuncture and education control groups.

Berman BM, Lao L, Langenberg P, Lee WL, Gilpin AM, Hochberg MC. Effectiveness of acupuncture as adjunctive therapy in osteoarthritis of the knee: a randomized, controlled trial. *Ann Intern Med*. 2004 Dec 21;141(12):901-10

In my opinion, this is a good piece of research for the following reasons:

- The authors had conducted several **pilot studies** and spent several years preparing for this definitive trial.
- The sample size was large and there was a proper **sample size calculation**.
- The patient group was clearly described.
- The treatment was appropriate (23 sessions).
- The follow up was sufficiently long.
- The **outcome measure** was adequate (a validated symptom score).
- All aspects of the trial were clearly described such that you or I could reproduce this study if we wanted.
- The conclusions were clear, cautious and correct.

Example 2

On 15th October 2002, six UK national newspapers reported that the supplement *'Coenzyme Q10 Holds Promise for Parkinson's Sufferers'*. Again, a US study was the cause.

BACKGROUND: Parkinson disease (PD) is a degenerative neurological disorder for which no treatment has been shown to slow the progression.

OBJECTIVE: To determine whether a range of dosages of coenzyme Q10 is safe and well tolerated and could slow the functional decline in PD.

DESIGN: Multicenter, randomized, parallel-group, placebo-controlled, double-blind, dosage-ranging trial.

SETTING: Academic movement disorders clinics.

PATIENTS: Eighty subjects with early PD who did not require treatment for their disability.

INTERVENTIONS: Random assignment to placebo or coenzyme Q10 at dosages of 300, 600, or 1200 mg/d.

MAIN OUTCOME MEASURE: The subjects underwent evaluation with the Unified Parkinson Disease Rating Scale (UPDRS) at the screening, baseline, and 1-, 4-, 8-, 12-, and 16-month visits. They were followed up for 16 months or until disability requiring treatment with levodopa had developed. The primary response variable was the change in the total score on the UPDRS from baseline to the last visit.

RESULTS: The adjusted mean total UPDRS changes were +11.99 for the placebo group, +8.81 for the 300-mg/d group, +10.82 for the 600-mg/d group, and +6.69 for the 1200-mg/d group. The P value for the primary analysis, a test for a linear trend between the dosage and the mean change in the total UPDRS score, was .09, which met our pre-specified criteria for a positive trend for the trial. A pre-specified, secondary analysis was the comparison of each treatment group with the placebo group, and the difference between the 1200-mg/d and placebo groups was significant (P = .04).

> **CONCLUSIONS:** Coenzyme Q10 was safe and well tolerated at dosages of up to 1200 mg/d. Less disability developed in subjects assigned to coenzyme Q10 than in those assigned to placebo, and the benefit was greatest in subjects receiving the highest dosage. Coenzyme Q10 appears to slow the progressive deterioration of function in PD, but these results need to be confirmed in a larger study.
>
> Shults CW, Oakes D, Kieburtz K, Beal MF, Haas R, Plumb S, Juncos JL, Nutt J, Shoulson I, Carter J, Kompoliti K, Perlmutter JS, Reich S, Stern M, Watts RL, Kurlan R, Molho E, Harrison M, Lew M; Parkinson Study Group. Effects of coenzyme Q10 in early Parkinson disease: evidence of slowing of the functional decline. *Arch Neurol*. 2002 Oct;59(10):1541-50

The study has a range of strengths.

- It tested not just the one but several dosages of Coenzyme Q10.
- Its sample size (80 patients) was not huge but adequate.
- The patient group was clearly described.
- The follow up was 16 months long.
- The primary outcome measure was appropriate (a validated symptom rating scale) and predefined.
- All other aspects of the methodology were clearly detailed.
- The conclusions were based on the findings (less disability in patients assigned Coenzyme Q10, **dose-effect relationship**, supplement was well tolerated) and drawn with the necessary caution (results should be checked in a larger study). The need for an independent confirmation of the results was stressed.

Examples of bad research

I find it somewhat embarrassing to 'name and shame'. Therefore, I have chosen two examples reported in UK daily papers to explain what some of the typical flaws of research are. Eccles and Hollinworth from London conducted a nurse-led **pilot study** of static magnets for healing leg ulcers.

Example 1

OBJECTIVE: To determine if UlcerCare, a specialised self-securing static magnetic device, can promote the healing of chronic leg ulcers.

METHOD: This double-blind placebo-controlled pilot study involved 26 patients with chronic leg ulcers, receiving care consistent with RCN guidelines, who were randomly allocated to receive either UlcerCare leg wrap (treatment) or an identical sham non-magnetic device (control). Wounds were assessed for 12 weeks at four weekly intervals using digital photography, Verge Videometer analysis and patient questionnaires to determine changes in ulcer size, level of pain and function.

RESULTS: Statistically significant reductions in ulcer measurement were noted in the treatment group when compared with the placebo group.

CONCLUSION: The results demonstrate a significant healing effect in the treatment group. A larger randomised controlled study is recommended to investigate the effects on ulcer-associated pain and quality of life.

Eccles NK, Hollinworth H. A pilot study to determine whether a static magnetic device can promote chronic leg ulcer healing. *J Wound Care*. 2005 Feb;14(2):64-7

The limitations of this study include:

- Small **sample size** (26 patients).
- Lack of **sample size calculation**
- **Randomisation** seems to have failed (patients in the experimental group had smaller ulcers to begin with).
- No firm conclusions could or should be drawn but the authors certainly did.

Example 2

Dryden et al from Winchester UK conducted a trial to test whether the efficacy of a 10% tea tree cream versus standard treatment for clearing MSRA colonisation.

Two topical MRSA eradication regimes were compared in hospital patients: a standard treatment included mupirocin 2% nasal ointment, chlorhexidine gluconate 4% soap, silver sulfadiazine 1% cream: versus a tea tree oil regimen, which included tea tree 10% cream, tea tree 5% body wash, both given for five days.

One hundred and fourteen patients received standard treatment and 56 (49%) were cleared of MRSA carriage. One hundred and ten received tea tree oil regimen and 46 (41%) were cleared.

There was no significant difference between treatment regimens (Fisher's exact test; P = 0.0286). Mupirocin was significantly more effective at clearing nasal carriage (78%) than tea tree cream (47%; P = 0.0001) but tea tree treatment was more effective than chlorhexidine or silver sulfadiazine at clearing superficial skin sites and skin lesions.

The tea tree preparations were effective, safe and well tolerated and could be considered in regimens for eradication of MRSA carriage.

Dryden MS, Dailly S, Crouch M. A randomized, controlled trial of tea tree topical preparations versus a standard topical regimen for the clearance of MRSA colonization. J Hosp Infect. 2004 Apr;56(4):283-6

The weaknesses of this study include:

- Many essential details of this study are poorly reported, thus its results cannot be reproduced by others.
- The results seem at odds with the conclusions drawn by the authors.
- It is impossible to judge whether the results are **generalisable**, i.e. transferable to other settings or patients.
- **Missing data** are not accounted for.
- It is unclear whether this study was designed as an **equivalence trial**.
- The conclusions are over-optimistic and the implications are not warranted by the data.

The language of research

The modern haematologist, instead of describing in English what he can see, prefers to describe in Greek what he can't (Richard Asher 1912-1969)

Anyone would be forgiven for finding the language of research less than accessible. When a researcher wants to tell his reader that he treated 50 patients with St John's Wort, he might state: '50 mild to moderate depressives were subjected to a regime of 3 x 900mg Hypericum perforatum extract per os'. It is hard to imagine a more pompous phraseology than that.

Sadly such language is often used in research papers. Here is a 'real life' example.

'To conclude, this randomized controlled study has demonstrated significant results relieving LBP in the elderly through the use of auriculotherapy with magnetic pellets'. Why not simply say, 'Our findings suggest that auricolotherapy with magnetic pellets is effective in controlling LBP'.

Precision

But don't blame the researchers. All they want to achieve is a precise terminology. To some the detached style may appear uncaring but, in my experience, this judgement would be wrong. The language of research serves foremost the purpose of accurately describing what is going on. A research paper must outline all aspects of the methodology in sufficient detail. The aim is to provide an account that enables the reader to repeat the experiment without any additional instructions.

More than one report needed

In medicine, one report on its own is rarely enough. This is not necessarily a sign of distrust – it is pure common sense. Before we change our clinical practice, we need to be sure that the findings are correct and reproducible. Every researcher knows that, even applying the highest level of rigour, many things can go wrong. Thus virtually any result could be at least partly due to chance or **bias**. Only when others have generated similar findings, can we be certain that we are dealing with something real and reliable. So precise language is of utmost importance.

Modern language

Luckily, the research community as a whole has somewhat changed its view on language in recent years. Many journals now encourage writers to use a more personal style, one which is more engaging, more attractive and easier to read. Consequently, the above statement might today read as follows:

'We recruited 50 patients who suffered from mild to moderate depression. We treated them with oral supplements containing St John's Wort (Hypericum perforation) at a daily dose of 3 x 900mg'.

The information is the same but it is clearly more accessible.

So, in case you are thinking of writing a research paper or article, don't be afraid of using a personal style. There is nothing wrong with using the first person. Use short, clear sentences that include all the relevant detail. Omit unnecessary ballast. And remember, that the main aim must be to convey exactly what is going on so that, whatever you are reporting, can be repeated and checked by others.

The structure of a research article

'Why did you start, what did you do, what answer did you get, and what does it mean anyway? That is a logical order of a scientific paper'
(Sir Austin Bradford-Hill, 1895-1991)

Over the years, a uniform structure of a research article has been universally accepted. An original research article is a communication reporting original data. Opinion pieces such as commentaries or editorials usually do not require a uniform structure. If you want to be able to understand published research, it seems essential that you are familiar with its standard structure.

This section is written as though I am giving instructions for writing a paper. Obviously not all readers will want to do that. But they will nevertheless profit from reading the section – it will show them what to expect of a research paper and what information can be found in which part of it.

The standard structure of an original paper

- Title/authors
- Abstract
- Introduction
- Methods
- Results
- Discussion
- Reference List
- Acknowledgments

Title
The title should be an exact and short description of the contents of the article. Ideally the reader should get a good impression whether this article is relevant for him by reading the title. Examples of good titles are:

- Ten cases of liver damage associated with kava (Piper methysticum) intake.
- A randomised trial of music therapy versus usual care reduces anxiety in hospitalized cancer patients.
- A survey of the prevalence of acupuncture-usage to reduce postoperative nausea.
- An interview study of the reasons for using dietary supplements in elderly arthritis sufferers.

Introduction

The introduction of a paper has the purpose of leading the reader into the subject at hand. It might address the following issues. Why is the topic important? What have previous studies shown? Why do the research now? What is your precise research question?

Method

The methods section should be an accurate account of what you have done. This is where precision is at its most important. It is the only section which enables other investigators to repeat your experiment. It is advisable to structure this section before writing it. In the case of a clinical trial, for instance, a useful structure could look like this.

Structure of methods section

- Full description of the patient population
  - Number
  - Age
  - Sex
  - Condition
  - Severity of condition
  - Length of condition
  - How it was verified?
- Setting, e.g. private practice, clinic, hospital.
- Treatments – both experimental and control
  - Nature of treatment
  - Dose of treatment
  - How frequently applied?
  - For how long?
  - By whom?
- Outcome measures
  - How were therapeutic success or failure verified, e.g. pain using a **visual analogue scale**?
  - Who did these measurements?
  - Did that person know about patients' **group allocation**?
  - Were there primary and secondary **outcome measures**?
  - When and how often were these measurements taken?

- Study design e.g. randomised, placebo-controlled double-blind trial.
  - Details about randomisation method.
  - Details about **blinding**.
- Statistical approach.
  - Type of analysis, e.g. intention to treat
  - Type of statistical test.
  - Was there a **power calculation**?
  - Was evaluator blinded?
- Approval of ethical committee?

Results

The results section should tell the reader clearly and concisely what you have found. Obviously this part too has to be complete and accurate. It is often useful to draw up tables presenting the numerical data. Sometimes it is helpful to include a graph, for instance, of the change over time in the primary outcome measure, e.g. decrease of pain in both groups.

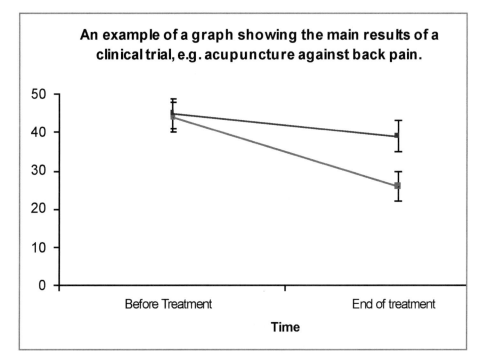

An example of a graph showing the main results of a clinical trial, e.g. acupuncture against back pain.

● + ■ = averages before and after treatment

I = variation of these averages, e.g. standard variation (see 000)

Horizontal axis (often called 'x axis') denotes time.

Vertical axis (often called 'y axis' may denote the primary **outcome measure** – in this case pain intensity.

Discussion

For first time writers, the discussion is usually the most challenging section. Here you need to briefly restate your main findings and subsequently put them into a more general context, e.g. of previous results from similar investigations.

You should also interpret the findings – e.g what do they mean for future healthcare? You might want to offer explanations as to the way the findings were brought about, e.g. do we understand how acupuncture reduces pain, or St. John's Wort alleviates depression?

Crucially, you must point out the strengths and weaknesses of your study. No investigation is absolutely flawless. Honesty requires that you alert your reader to the limitations of your work. Sometimes it is helpful to provide suggestions for future research. Most studies open new questions and you might point the reader as to how you think they can be answered.

Finally you should come to a final conclusion. It is crucial that these are not extrapolations but strictly reflect the results you have produced; after all you are seeking the 'truth' not trying to prove a point.

References

The reference list must include the most important previous papers in this area. If should be up-to-date and must back up all major statements in the text. For instance, if you say 'previous research has shown that postoperative pain can be effectively treated with acupuncture', you need to cite the article(s) that demonstrate this fact.

Acknowledgements

In the acknowledgements you might thank those people who have helped you, if they are not already included in the list of authors. You must also disclose any financial support or other potential conflicts of interest.

A critical appraisal

Learning without thinking is useless; thinking without learning is dangerous (Confucius 551-478 BC)

Critical appraisal is the analysis of evidence in a systematic, conscious and explicit fashion. In a way, it is a summary of much of what has been stated on the previous pages. For interpreting research papers, critical appraisal is an essential tool. One way of using it is by asking several straight forward questions.

1. Is there a clear research question?

The importance of this cannot be over-emphasised. The value of any research project crucially hinges on a concise and clear research question. In the absence of such a question, the reader encounters difficulties in understanding essential elements of the study.

2. Is the research question important?

If a piece of research is not important, it should probably have not been conducted in the first place. But the issue is, of course, complex. What is important to one person might not be so to another. What does 'important' mean anyway? It should mean that the results of that project have some potential for improving future healthcare. The findings therefore should matter not just to you and your friends, but to a sizable group of people. Classical examples of important questions are those that concern populations or relate to serious healthcare problems.

It is perhaps easier to think of unimportant research questions. Two examples may suffice.

- Is urine-therapy effective for alopecia?
  Urine-therapy is not used by many people. There is no suggestion that it might be helpful for hair loss. Moreover, alopecia is not a life-threatening condition.

- Does therapeutic touch prevent heart attacks?
  Both heart attacks and therapeutic touch are prevalent. Yet, this research question is not biologically plausible. Today we understand fairly well what brings about heart attacks, and therapeutic touch is not likely to interfere with these mechanisms. Lastly a prevention trial of this nature would require a very large **sample size** and a long **follow-up**. It is unrealistic to think that such a study could be feasible.

Plausibility and feasibility

Two further criteria are thus relevant: plausibility and feasibility. As research funds will always be limited, it makes sense to tackle those questions which have the greatest possibility of generating results which would be of value to others. This means implausible treatments are not usually top of the list. The problem here is that plausibility is not a well-defined concept. Some opponents of CAM, for instance, would argue that this whole area is biologically implausible. On the other hand, I am sure that many nurses would believe that therapeutic touch is not implausible.

Feasibility is an important concept. If a project is not 'doable', it cannot normally be a priority. If the research question is impossible to tackle, everything that follows is likely to be meaningless.

3. What do we already know?

If there were already dozens of rigorous trials on the subject in question and all showed similar results, it makes little sense to conduct a **pilot study**. If the previous studies were flawed, however, it would be reasonable to conduct a trial that overcomes these limitations. If we know nothing about a given subject, it might be unwise to conduct a large-scale trial. In this case, it would probably be better to do small explorative studies which eventually might guide us towards conducting a well-planned, definitive trial.

Critical appraisal therefore benefits from sound knowledge of the subject area. It may thus include the study of previous research in order to place the current results in the right context.

4. Is the study design adequate?

As I have stressed before, there are no inherently adequate or inadequate study designs. A study is adequately designed if it can answer the research question at hand and minimises bias. In the case of the above-formulated question (massage for back pain), this objective is best achieved by a randomised, clinical study. Whatever the research question is, it is crucial that the study minimises **bias**. Biased studies tend to generate **false positive results** and are therefore likely to mislead us.

5. Are the methods fully described?

A hallmark of good research is reproducibility. Thus any study must be reported in such a way that the reader could replicate it. When critically appraising a published research project, one should constantly ask oneself when reading the methods section, do the authors provide sufficient details for another person to reproduce this study in exactly the same way they conducted it?

But there are other important points to consider.

The **sample size** should be sufficient to detect a statistically significant effect if there is one. A **power calculation** is required which determines the sample size. In reports of clinical trials, are baseline demographic characteristics and baseline values of the outcome measures comparable?

Were the experimenter, assessor and/or subjects blinded to treatment allocation? The failure to have an appropriate **sham** control and proper blinding can produce **false positive results**. It is useful to ask how the patients' expectations have been managed. Is the design such that they are likely to have been disappointed by allocation to the control procedure and encouraged by allocation to the test intervention? We all know how importantly such sentiments can influence a clinical outcome.

6. What are the results?

Critical appraisal of the results of quantitative research is only possible if they are provided numerically in full detail. Describing the results in words or graphically is not enough. Ideally the reader should be in a position to recalculate the statistics on the primary outcome measures. For this, the minimum requirements are **group averages** and a measure of their variation.

Controlled trials have the purpose of comparing changes in outcomes generated by the experimental intervention with those generated by the control intervention. Therefore we need between group comparisons – before and after (**intra-group**) differences are misleading in the context of controlled studies.

It is advisable to run 'reality checks' on the results. Ask yourself questions such as, is this finding plausible? Could it be explained by other factors? Is it corroborated by other results?

7. Is the discussion adequate?

In critically appraising the discussion, we might ask ourselves, do the authors put their results into the context of all previous data on the subject, or are they selective in citing only evidence that supports their own findings? Are their interpretations all the conceivable interpretations, or are there other ones which they fail to mention? Are the authors capable of criticising their own research? Do they constructively lead the reader to the type of research that might address the questions which remain currently unanswered? Do the authors provide reasonable guidance as to what we should do with this evidence in clinical practice?

8. Are the conclusions correct?

Authors often over-interpret their own results and draw conclusions that are not actually based on the data they have generated. Over-optimistic interpretation of the results is particularly common in CAM. Critical appraisal should evaluate whether the research question is adequately addressed by the trial methodology and properly reflected in the conclusion. All elements of a research paper should be congruent with each other.

9. Are there conflicts of interest?

The most obvious source of conflicts of interest arises through sponsorship. We know, for instance, that commercially funded trials tend to generate more positive results than studies which do not have such support. Therefore funding has to be disclosed – even the fact that there was no external financial support should be mentioned.

In CAM, physiotherapy or nursing, there are relatively few commercial interests – but plenty of non-commercial ones. These are very rarely disclosed. Arguably it matters whether the authors of an acupuncture trial earn their living through acupuncture, are officers of an acupuncture society, or are long-term advocates of acupuncture. Such people are, of course, not incapable of conducting good research. But these 'interests' must be laid open.

Common flaws in research

By far the most common and easily avoidable flaw in medical research is drawing inaccurate conclusions. The conclusions of a piece of research are only valid if they directly follow from the data. If not, they are extrapolations which are based not on fact but on wishful thinking.

Another frequent mistake is the fact that studies are often too small to generate definitive results. This is understandable because the size of an investigation determines its cost. As research funds are scarce, investigators are often forced to be miserly with the sample size. In the end, this can lead to unreliable results, e.g. no effect was observed not because the treatment was ineffective but because there were not enough patients in the trial, and the statistics therefore had to fail.

Common flaws in research studies

Within my team of researchers, we conducted a little survey. Each of us had to name those flaws in research studies which occur most often. The two mentioned above were clear 'favourites'. Here are, in descending order, other frequent drawbacks.

- Reporting of 'within-group' or 'before-after' (**intra-group**) differences in controlled clinical trials. The whole point of having a **control group** in a clinical trial is comparing its results to those of the **experimental group**. Before-after differences can be brought about by the condition getting better on its own. This factor is eliminated when we compare the results of the experimental group to those of the control group.
- No or incorrect **randomisation** in clinical trials.
- No or inadequate **blinding** in clinical trials.
- Incongruence of aims and methods of a research project.
- Incomplete description of the research methods.
- Inadequate comparator intervention in controlled clinical trials.
- No pre-defined primary **outcome measure** in clinical trials.

CHAPTER 3 — DISSECTING RESEARCH PAPERS: TWO EXAMPLES

In this section I have selected two of my own examples of research, a clinical trial and a systematic review, to illustrate the principles of research with a view of developing your understanding of published research. Of course, two examples are not enough to achieve this aim, but perhaps they give valuable clues and can get you started in reading and understanding research papers.

Paper 1

This first article is a clinical trial of flower remedies for reduction of exam stress (Perfusion 1999, 12:440–46). Its introduction essentially describes what flower remedies are and ends with a concise statement about the aim of the study:

The aim of this trial was to test whether Five Flower Remedy® (also marketed as Rescue Remedy®), one of the most popular BFRs, is efficacious in reducing examination anxiety in university students.

(BFRs) – Bach flower remedies.

Subjects and methods[1]

Subjects[2]
University students were found through a series of advertising activities and were given a verbal and written explanation of the study.[3] Interested volunteers were screened according to predefined inclusion/exclusion criteria. The inclusion criteria[4] included current registration at the University of Exeter, age between 18 to 65 years, and registration to undertake university examinations between May

1. This is the start of the 'methods' section of this paper.

2. Sometimes it is clearer to use subheadings within the 'methods' section.

3. The methods of recruiting volunteers can be important, for instance, if you wanted to replicate this study.

4. It is essential that the inclusion/ exclusion criteria are explicit.

to July 1998. All volunteers indicated that they experienced some degree of anxiety or 'exam nerves' before taking examinations.

Exclusion criteria[5] included pregnancy, concurrent treatment for depression, concurrent use of antipsychotic medication, anxiolytic agents, other flower remedies, and/or other psychotherapeutic approaches to anxiety relief.

Sample size calculation[6]

Sample size was calculated using the approximate formula (Senn 1997) for sample size:

$$n = 2 \, (Z_{\alpha/2} + Z_{\beta})^2 \, \sigma^2 / {}_{\Delta}^2 \; [7]$$

such that the value of α was set at 0.05, the value β selected was 0.2 to allow the detection of any significant differences with 80% power, with σ (the standard deviation) estimated as 11.41 (Spielberger 1983) and a clinically relevant difference (Δ) of 6 using data from previous studies (Spielberger 1983). This yielded an approximate sample size of 41 per group.

Randomization and concurrent controls

Volunteers were randomised using block randomisation[8] (block size of four) to receive either Five Flower Remedy or an indistinguishable placebo. Both[9] were prepared by Healing Herbs. Five Flower Remedy is the rescue remedy combination according to Dr Bach containing the following flower essences: Prunus cerasifera, Clematis vitalba, Impatiens glandulifera, Helianthemum nummularium and Ornithogalum umbellatum. Verum vials were prepared by adding 2 drops of Five-Flower essence to 10 mls of brandy (40% alcohol by volume).[10] Placebo remedy was prepared in a similar manner with the exclusion of addition of Five-Flower essence. Placebo and verum vials were separately packed in cardboard boxes and posted to the Department of Complementary Medicine, University of Exeter where they were received by the study pharmacist who independently assigned a study number to each bottle.[11]

Dosing regimen

Participants were instructed to take one to four doses of their assigned remedy per day and to follow this regimen between Day 1 and Day 7 of the trial period. One dose (as recommended by the manufacturer) comprised 4 drops of remedy in a small glass of water to be sipped frequently over an unspecified period of time. Benefit

5. It would create a false negative result if one treated people for a condition they don't have.

6. It is important that study's sample size is large enough to detect an effect. If it is too small, a false negative result might be generated.

7. Statistics can be complex and it is advisable to recruit a statistician for it. I too would use a statistician to define these.

8. To simply state that 'allocation was by randomisation' may not be enough – the precise method of randomisation can be important.

9. Randomisation has to be done by someone not directly involved in the running of the trial.

10. If anyone wants to repeat this study, he or she should be able to replicate the treatment. So, a full description is necessary.

11. It is important that the trialists were unable to guess which treatments were verum and which placebo.

is claimed to be derived from small, regular use rather than by the volume of remedy that is taken.[12]

Measurement of anxiety

The 40-item Spielberger State-Trait Anxiety Inventory (STAI) was the primary outcome measure used to quantify anxiety (Spielberger 1983) experienced by the participants.[13] It comprises two separate scales namely, the State anxiety score which aims to quantify the extent to which an emotional state exists at a given moment in time at a particular level of intensity and the Trait anxiety score which refers to relatively stable individual differences in anxiety-proneness. The stronger the anxiety Trait, the more probable that the individual will experience more intense elevations in State anxiety in a threatening situation. This two-component self-evaluation questionnaire was administered three times throughout the investigation: at induction, 7 days before the examination specified as likely to cause most anxiety to the student, the night before examination and after the examination. Visual analogue scales[14] with polar opposite concepts (**no anxiety** and **worst imaginable anxiety**) were used as the secondary outcome measure to allow the determination of daily anxiety scores.

Adverse effects[15] data and compliance[16]

Participants were asked to indicate the number of doses (0 to a maximum of 4) used per day and were invited to detail any perceived adverse effects during the course of the investigation.

Follow-up[17]

Reminder letters were sent to participants who had not returned their study documents at the expected date of return. One month later, all non-responders were sent a short multiple choice questionnaire in order to remind those who had completed but had still not returned the study documents to do so and to ascertain the reasons for non-completion.

Ethical approval[18] and consent[19]

Ethical approval was obtained from the local ethics committee (South and West Local Research Ethics Committee, Department of Medical Affairs, Royal Devon & Exeter Hospital, Barrack Road, Exeter, EX2 5DW). A clinical trial certificate was deemed unnecessary by the Medicines Control Agency. Written informed consent was obtained from all participants.

12. It would be irrelevant to test a treatment which nobody claims to be effective.

13. Outcome measures should be validated and relevant to the condition treated.

14. Visual analogue scales are popular for quantifying subjective symptoms.

15. Adverse effects are undesired occurrences during the trial period. They may or may not be caused by the treatment.

16. Checking for compliance may be important: if a remedy is not administered, it cannot be effective. Poor compliance might therefore create a false negative result.

17. This describes the length of the study period.

18. All research on humans or animals requires approval from an independent ethics committee.

19. Informed consent is an ethical imperative.

Statistical analysis

Blinded data analysis was carried out using SPSS version 8.0 for Windows. P values[20] of less than 0.05 were considered statistically significant. Analysis of covariance[21] was used to produce a measure of anxiety which is adjusted by baseline in such a way that the result is uncorrelated with the baseline.[22] The analysis of covariance estimator also has the advantage that its variance is generally lower than that using raw outcomes or change scores. The linear contrast variable was calculated from daily VAS score for anxiety, designed to isolate the slope of any underlying linear trend. Using the following equation to model the linear relationship, $VAS_{LC}=3(V_7)+2(V_6)+(V_5)-(V_3)-2(V_2)-3(V_t)$ where V is the VAS score for each day (indicated by the subscript number), V_4 having a zero coefficient, then assuming that if $V_t=a+b_t+error$ where V is the VAS score, a is the fixed constant, b is the slope of the linear relationship and t is the time point, then $VAS_{LC}=28_b+error$. Values are expressed as $VAS_{LC}/28$ in order to give units as mm per day (mmd^{-1}).[21]

Results

Of the 100 subjects who were recruited and randomized, 51 were assigned to Five Flower Remedy (19 men, 32 women) and 49 to placebo (14 men, 35 women).[23] 45% of the participants completed the study; 21 subjects in the experimental group and 24 subjects in the placebo group (Fig. 1). The relative percentages of each gender completing remained comparatively constant within the groups. Of those subjects who did not complete the study, three withdrew,[24] 39 were lost of follow-up and 13 gave reasons for non-participation[25] (Fig. 1). Eight of those non-completing subjects who gave reasons for non-participation took the assigned remedy for a number of days (Five Flower Remedy 1.80±0.84, placebo 2.00±1.73; two-tailed t-test P=0.099) before terminating. Reasons for non-completion in this group included forgetting to take remedy (4 subjects), using all the remedy before 7 days (1 subject) not finding remedies palatable (1 subject), breaking remedy bottle (one subject), perceiving an adverse effect (1 subject). Of those who reported that they did not take the remedy at all, 60% (3 subjects) reported that they had forgotten to take the remedy, 20% (1 subject) reported that the remedy was not palatable and 20% (one subject) perceived the participant burden to be too high. Table 1 compares the baseline characteristics of participants and non-participants.[22] The average age of those recruits who went on to complete the study was very similar to those who did not complete.

20. p-values indicate the likelihood with which a result might have occurred by chance.

21. Statistics can be complex – it is best to consult a specialist.

22. Baseline data are the characteristics of volunteers at entry into the study.

23. Because allocation was by randomisation, numbers can be uneven.

24. Withdrawals are volunteers who had to be removed from the study e.g. because of non-compliance.

25. Dropouts are volunteers who simply leave the study without permission.

Participants reported that they experienced examination nerves to an equal degree between groups (Pearson two-sided chi-square p=0.378).[20] Similar proportions of participants and non-participants were smokers (Pearson two-sided chi-square p=0.145)[20] but of those who did smoke, non-participants reported greater cigarette consumption (two-tailed t-test p=0.006).[20] Equal proportions of participants and non-participants reported that they consumed alcohol (Pearson two-sided chi-square p=0.94).[26] However, reported alcohol intake was greater in non-participants (two-tailed t-test p=0.035). Reported frequency of exercise session[26] lasting more than 20 min was comparable between groups (Pearson two-sided chi-square p=0.163). Both components of the STAI were similar (state anxiety, participants 43.4±11.2 non-participants 43.7±11.2; two-tailed t-test p=0.884; trait anxiety, participants 41.4±11.2 non-participants 41.8±10.1; two-tailed t-test p=0.844). Concurrent non-parametric tests (Mann-Whitney U tests) were found to agree with all the above parametric tests.[27]

Table 2[28] compares the baseline characteristics of the experimental and the control groups. Similar proportions of men and women in both groups completed the study; these were broadly representative of the proportions upon recruitment. Within the experimental group, 14 were male (31%)[29] and 31 (69%) were female and within the placebo group, 19 (35%) were male and 36 (65%) were female. No significant differences between or within groups were found for mean[30] age of participants and no interactions between the main effects were identified (two-way ANOVA p=0.566, p=0.138 and p=0.456 respectively). Year of study and reported 'examination nerves' seem similar across groups and gender, as do the proportions of smokers and consumers of alcohol. Reported number of exercise sessions per week was not significantly different between or within groups and no interaction between these factors was identified (two-way ANOVA p=0.718, p=0.319 and p=0.977 respectively). Reporting of situational anxiety (State at time 0) was not found to differ significantly[31] according to group allocation or gender of the participant. Again no interaction between the main effects was found (two-way ANOVA p=0.936, p=0.110 and 0.763 respectively). A main effect for gender was identified for reported trait anxiety upon enrolment. When asked to **describe how you generally feel** (trait anxiety score), men consistently scored lower than women (Trait at time 0) with no statistical significance for group allocation or interaction (two-way ANOVA p=0.828, p=0.043

26. This could be an important confounder and confounders should always be reported openly.

27. The reason for using randomisation is that it renders both groups comparable.

28. Numerical, complex data are best presented in table format (omitted here).

29. Sometimes it is best to present numbers both as absolute figures and percentages.

30. Mean is the sum of all data divided by the amount of single data points.

31. This term signifies a 95% chance that the effect is real.

and p=0.564 respectively). Table 3[28] compares the treatment outcomes between the experimental and the control groups. Self-reports of dose of remedy taken were not found to significantly differ according to treatment group allocation or gender of the participant. A statistically significant interaction was identified which indicated that the men in the placebo group took significantly fewer doses of their allocated remedy (two-way ANOVA p=0.014). Men were found to report significantly lower levels of anxiety eight days before the examination (State 1 score) identified as most likely to cause increased anxiety as measured by the State component of the STAI (two-way ANOVA p=0.001). No statistically significant differences between the experimental and placebo groups were identified for the State anxiety score measured on the evening before the examination (State 2 score). Analysis of covariance was carried out on the State 2 score using State 1 as a covariate since men and women evaluated their level of anxiety differently 8 days before examination. (All other logical covariates were fitted in the model but no further benefit was gained by their addition.) This analysis did not alter the statistical significance found for group, sex or the interaction term (ANOVA p=0.641, 0.981 and 0.812 respectively). No statistically significant differences were found for the mean of the daily VAS scores. The linear contrast variable for the weekly VAS reports was not found to be significantly different between or within groups.[32] Daily mean VAS scores along with the standard error of the means are presented in Table 3 and Figure 2.[33] No significant differences between the men and women in the experimental and placebo groups were found at the beginning of the study period. Men were found to report lower anxiety as measured on the VAS scale than women on days 1 and 2 of the study (two-way ANOVA p=0.011 and p=0.048 respectively). On day 3 participants taking the active remedy reported significantly less anxiety on the VAS scale than those in the placebo group (two-way ANOVA p=0.041). No other statistically significant effects were observed over the study period. Correlation between anxiety and dose taken shows no clear relationship. This was investigated according to treatment allocation for all participating students. Three subjects from both the verum and the placebo group reported a total of five different perceived adverse effects.[15] Those reported in the verum group included headaches (two subjects – one withdrew from the study after three days as a result) and skin eruptions. The reported adverse effects in subjects taking

32. In plain language: the verum did not produce effects that were different from placebo.

33. Sometimes data can be visualised in graphs for more clarity.

the placebo included vomiting before the examination, hayfever symptoms and depressive mood (subject withdrew as a result).[34]

Paper 2

The second paper is a systematic review of clinical trials of horse chestnut seed extract to treat chronic venous insufficiency. It was published on the Cochrane database and updated in 2007 (www.cochrane.org/reviews/). The article starts with a title (Horse chestnut seed extract for chronic venous insufficiency) a table of contents, a structured abstract, a plain language summary and continues with the article proper.

Background[1]

Chronic venous insufficiency (CVI) is one of the commonest conditions afflicting humans. About 10-15% of men and 20-25% of women present signs and symptoms consistent with the diagnosis of CVI, indicating that being female is an important risk factor, as well as age, geographical location and race (Callam 1992; Callam 1994). This condition is characterised by chronic inadequate drainage of venous blood and venous hypertension, which results in leg oedema (swelling), dermatosclerosis (hardening of the skin) and feelings of pain, fatigue and tenseness in the lower extremities (Spraycar 1995). Patients often require hospitalization and surgery of, for instance, symptomatic varicose veins (London 2000; Michaels 2000). Mechanical compression is the treatment of choice for this condition (Partsch 1991). However, compression therapy, for example, using compression stockings often causes discomfort and has been associated with poor compliance. Oral drug treatment is therefore an attractive option.[2]

Horse chestnut (*Aesculus hippocastanum L.*) has traditionally been used as a herbal remedy for treating CVI (Bombardelli 1996). The seed extract of *AesculushippocastanumL.* (HCSE) contains escin, a triterpenic saponin, as its active component (Guillaume 1994; Lorenz 1960; Schrader 1995). Escin has been shown to inhibit the activity of elastase and hyaluronidase, two enzymes involved in proteoglycan degradation (Facino 1995). The accumulation of leucocytes (white blood cells) in CVI-affected limbs (Moyses 1987; Thomas 1988) and subsequent activation and release of such enzymes (Sarin 1993) is considered to be an important pathophysiological mechanism of CVI. It has been suggested that HCSE works by preventing leucocyte activation (Facino 1995). However, regardless of the postulated mechanism of action, the most important questions are whether it is safe and efficacious for treating patients with CVI.[3]

Objectives[4]

To review the evidence from rigorous clinical trials assessing the efficacy and safety of HCSE versus placebo, or reference therapy, for the symptomatic treatment of CVI.

Method[5]

Criteria for considering studies for this review[6]

Types of studies

Randomised, controlled trials (RCTs), i.e. trials with a randomized generation of allocation sequences. Studies assessing acute effects only were excluded. No restrictions regarding the language of publication were imposed (Egger 1997).

Types of participants

Studies were included if participants were patients with CVI. Studies that did not use adequate diagnostic criteria (e.g.Widmer 1978) were excluded.

Types of intervention

Trials were included if they compared oral preparations containing HCSE as the only active component (mono-preparation) with placebo or reference therapy. Trials assessing HCSE as one of several active components in a combination preparation or as a part of a combination treatment were excluded.[7]

Types of outcome measures[8]

Trials using clinical outcome measures were included. The outcome measures were CVI-related symptoms (e.g. leg pain, pruritus (itching), oedema (swelling)), leg volume, circumference at ankle and calf, and adverse events as reported in the included trials. Studies focusing exclusively on physiological parameters were excluded.

3. The introduction continues to describe the treatment under scrutiny. The average healthcare professional is unlikely to know about this herbal remedy – had this article been published in a journal for herbalists, this would probably be redundant.

4. It is important to provide a very clear statement about the aim of the paper. The best place for this is usually at the end of the introduction.

5. This is where the 'methods' section starts – in most journals this would be indicated with a heading 'methods'.

6. This information is essential for anyone who might want to replicate this research.

7. If more than one herbal medicine is administered, it would be difficult to decide which caused the effect.

8. It seemed important to include symptoms, which are important to patients, and signs, which can often be measured more objectively.

Search methods for identification of studies[9]

See: Peripheral Vascular Diseases Group methods used in reviews.

We searched the Cochrane Peripheral Vascular Diseases Specialised Register (last searched October 2005), the Cochrane Central Register of Controlled Trials (CENTRAL) (*The Cochrane Library* Issue 3, 2005), AMED (inception to July 2005) and Phytobase (inception to January 2001, not operational any longer). The search strategy and terms used to search CENTRAL are given in Table 01. Search terms used for AMED and Phytobase are given in Table 02.

The Specialised Trials Register of the PVD Group has been constructed from regular electronic searches of MEDLINE (January 1966 to date), EMBASE (January 1980 to date), and CENTRAL (current Issue of *The Cochrane Library*) and through handsearching 38 relevant journals and numerous conference proceedings. Relevant trials are entered into the Register. The full list of journals and conference proceedings, as well as the search strategies for the electronic databases, are described in the 'Search strategies for the identification of studies' section within the editorial information about the Cochrane Peripheral Vascular Diseases Group.

In addition, manufacturers of HCSE preparations and experts on the subject were contacted and asked to contribute published and unpublished material. Furthermore, our own files were scanned. The bibliographies of the studies thus retrieved were searched for further trials.

Methods of the review

Max Pittler and Edzard Ernst independently screened and selected trials for inclusion, assessed their methodological quality and extracted data. Disagreements at any of these stages were resolved by discussion.[10]

Selection of trials

Trials were selected according to the criteria outlined above under Types of Studies.

Methodological quality[11]

Methodological quality was evaluated using the scoring system developed by Jadad (Jadad 1996). This scale quantifies the likelihood of bias inherent in the trials based on the reporting of randomisation, blinding and withdrawals. Trials are awarded points on a scale of one to five, where five denotes trial reporting suggesting relatively high quality and low risk of bias, and one

9. In order to create the most reliable overall picture, it is essential that all studies are included. The search strategy has to be thorough and, for reasons of transparency, it should be described in full detail.

10. Usually it is preferable to have two independent reviewers extracting the data. This minimises the likelihood of error.

11. Studies of low methodological quality are open to bias and therefore can produce misleading results. For interpreting conflicting data, it is essential to account for the scientific rigour of the primary data.

denotes trial reporting suggesting relatively low quality and high risk of bias. Only RCTs were included in this review – independent of their quality score. Trials were also given a score for concealment of treatment allocation, where A = clearly concealed, B = unclear if concealed, C = clearly not concealed, and D = concealment of allocation was not used.

Data extraction[12]

The following data were extracted:

1. Participant characteristics: age, gender.

2. Methods used: randomisation, double-blinding, concealment of treatment allocation, description of drop outs.

3. Interventions: oral preparations containing HCSE as the only active component (mono-preparation), compared with placebo or comparator medication(s).

4. Outcome measures: CVI-related symptoms (e.g. leg pain, pruritus, oedema), leg volume, circumference at ankle and calf, and adverse events.

Statistical analysis[13]

Statistical pooling of trial data was performed. However, the lack of a common outcome measure and the heterogeneity of instruments used limits the conclusiveness of these analyses.

Statistical analysis was performed using RevMan Analyses 1.0.4. It uses the inverse of the variance to assign a weight to the mean of the within-study treatment effect. For most studies, however, the information was insufficient. The Cochrane Collaboration suggests to impute the variance of the change by assuming a correlation factor between pre-intervention and post-intervention values. The variance of the change was imputed using a correlation factor of 0.4, which was then used to assign a weight to the mean of the within-study treatment effect. Data-pooling of continuous data was performed using the weighted mean difference; for dichotomous data the odds ratio was used. Summary estimates of the treatment effect were calculated using a random effects model. The chi-square test for heterogeneity tested whether the distribution of the results was compatible with the assumption that intertribal differences were attributable to chance variation alone.

Sensitivity analyses to test the robustness of the main analysis will be performed in future if more data become available.

12. It is important that researchers pre-define the type of data they want to extract. Usually this is done already in the protocol of the project. It can be relevant to define the best outcome measures in a team that includes patients.

13. This can be highly specialised and usually it is advisable to consult a statistician.

Description of studies[14]

Twenty-nine randomised controlled clinical trials assessing oral mono-preparations containing HCSE were identified. This included two unpublished trials (Cloarec 1992; Diehm 2000).[15] Seventeen trials met the above mentioned inclusion criteria (Cloarec 1992; Diehm 1992; Diehm 1996a; Diehm 2000; Erdlen 1989; Erler 1991; Friederich 1978; Kalbeisch 1989; Koch 2002; Lohr 1986; Morales 1993; Neiss 1976; Pilz 1990; Rehn 1996; Rudofsky 1986; Steiner 1986; Steiner 1990a). Twelve trials were excluded: three were duplicate publications (Pauschinger 1987; Steiner 1990b; Steiner 1991); seven tested HCSE as a component in combination preparations or combination treatments (Boehm 1989; Coninx 1974; Dols 1987; Dustmann 1984; Hirsch 1982; Neumann-Mangoldt '79; Zuccarelli 1986); and two focused exclusively on physiological parameters (Bisler 1986; Lochs 1974).[16]

Of the seventeen trials included in the review, ten were placebo-controlled; two compared HCSE against reference treatment with compression stockings and placebo (Diehm 1996a; Diehm 2000); four were controlled against reference medication with O-,-hydroxyethyl rutosides (HR) (Erdlen 1989; Erler 1991; Kalbeisch 1989; Rehn 1996) and one was controlled against medication with pycnogenol (Koch 2002). All of these studies administered HCSE in capsules, permitting the preparation of adequate placebos. In all trials the extract was standardised to escin which is the main active constituent of HCSE.[17]

Methodological quality[18]

All the included RCTs except one (Koch 2002) were double-blinded. They scored at least one out of five points on the Jadad scale (Jadad 1996). Three trials scored A and the remaining fourteen trials scored B for the method of allocation concealment. Key data from the included trials, including scores for quality and allocation concealment, are presented in the Table 'Characteristics of included studies'.[19]

Results

The majority of the included studies diagnosed the patients according to the classification by Widmer (Widmer 1978). Fourteen trials reported inclusion criteria for CVI patients relating to this classification. Eighty-two percent of the participants in these trials were categorised into CVI stages I, II or I-II. Three trials, comprising 22% of the total number of participants did not refer to this

14. In most journals, this would be the beginning of the 'results' section – but here the structure is slightly different.

15. It can be important to retrieve even those studies that have not been published. This emphasises the importance of a thorough search strategy (see above)

16. For the purpose of repeatability, it is essential to name those studies that were found but had to be excluded and provide the reasons why.

17. If we fail to define the treatment as closely as possible, the findings become uninterpretable.

18. As mentioned above quality matters importantly. This is best expressed numerically rather than verbally (e.g. good or satisfactory).

19. The results need to be provided in full detail. Usually this is easiest in table format.

classification.[20] Overall, the included placebo-controlled trials suggested an improvement in the CVI related symptoms of leg pain, oedema and pruritus.

Leg pain[21]

Leg pain was assessed in seven placebo-controlled trials (Cloarec 1992; Friederich 1978; Lohr 1986; Morales 1993; Neiss 1976; Rudofsky 1986; Steiner 1990a). Six studies (n = 543)[22] reported a statistically significant reduction (P < 0.05)[23] of leg pain on various measurement scales in participants treated with HCSE compared with placebo, while another reported an improvement compared with baseline (Steiner 1990a). One study (Cloarec 1992), reported adequate data (i.e. data that are included within RevMan Analyses 1.0.4 and can be used for meta-analysis) assessed on a 100 mm VAS, suggesting a weighted mean difference (WMD) of 42.40 mm (95% confidence interval (CI) 34.90 to 49.90). Other studies which compared HCSE with HR (Kalbeisch 1989), pycnogenol (Koch 2002) or compression (Diehm 2000) reported no significant intergroup differences for leg pain or a symptom score including leg pain.

Oedema

Oedema was assessed in six placebo-controlled trials (Cloarec 1992; Friederich 1978; Lohr 1986; Morales 1993; Neiss 1976; Steiner 1990a). Four trials (n = 461) reported a statistically significant reduction of oedema in participants treated with HCSE compared with placebo, whilst one (Steiner 1990a) reported an improvement compared with baseline. One study (Cloarec 1992) reported adequate data suggesting a WMDof 40.10 mm (95% CI 31.60 to 48.60) in favour of HCSE assessed on a 100 mm VAS.[24] Another study (Koch 2002) reported that HCSE was inferior to pycnogenol, whereas a further trial (Diehm 2000) reported no significant differences for a score including the symptom oedema compared with compression. Oedema provocation before and after treatment with HCSE revealed oedema protective effects (Erler 1991).

Pruritus

Pruritus was assessed in eight placebo-controlled trials (Diehm 1992; Friederich 1978; Lohr 1986; Morales 1993; Neiss 1976; Rudofsky 1986; Steiner 1986; Steiner 1990a). Four trials (n = 407) suggested a statistically significant reduction of pruritus in participants treated with HCSE compared with placebo (P < 0.05). Two trials (Steiner 1986; Steiner 1990a) suggested a statistically significant[25] difference in favour of HCSE compared with baseline (P

20. If we did not know what type of patients were treated, we would have great difficulties in interpreting the results.

21. Often it is advisable to report the results according to specific outcome measures.

22. The sample size is often depicted as 'n'.

23. The p-value gives a measure of probability that the result is real and not due to chance.

24. Visual analogue scales are often used as outcome measures to quantify subjective symptoms.

< 0.05). Another trial (Kalbeisch 1989), which compared HCSE with HR, but failed to include a placebo group,[26] seemed to corroborate these findings. A further trial (Diehm 2000) reported no significant differences for a score[27] including the symptom pruritus compared with compression.

Leg volume[28]

Leg volume was assessed in seven placebo-controlled trials (Diehm 1992; Diehm 1996a; Diehm 2000; Lohr 1986; Rudofsky 1986; Steiner 1986; Steiner 1990a). All of these studies used water displacement plethysmometry to measure this outcome. Meta-analysis[29] of six trials (Diehm 1992; Diehm 1996a; Diehm 2000 ; Rudofsky 1986; Steiner 1986; Steiner 1990a; n = 502) suggested a WMD of 32.1ml (95% CI[30] 13.49 to 50.72) in favour of HCSE compared with placebo (pooled standardised mean difference 0.34; 95% CI 0.15 to 0.52). One trial (Rehn 1996) reported findings suggesting that HCSE was equivalent[31] to HR, and another (Diehm 1996a, n = 194) suggested that it may be as efficacious as treatment with compression stockings (WMD -2.90 ml; 95% CI - 30.42 to 24.62).

Significant beneficial effects for CVI patients were reported in trials which administered HCSE standardised to 100-150 mg escin daily.[32] Three studies, using 100 mg escin daily, reported a statistically significant reduction of mean[33] leg volume after two weeks of treatment compared with placebo (P ò 0.01) (Rudofsky 1986; Steiner 1986; Steiner 1990a). Persistence of treatment effects was suggested by one study (Rehn 1996). At the end of a six-week follow-up[34] period mean leg volume was similar to post-treatment values.

Circumference

Circumference at calf and ankle was assessed in seven placebo-controlled trials (Cloarec 1992; Diehm 1992; Lohr 1986; Pilz 1990; Rudofsky 1986; Steiner 1986; Steiner 1990a). Five studies (n = 172) suggested a statistically significant reduction at the ankle, and three (n = 112) at the calf in favour of HCSE compared with placebo. At the ankle, meta-analysis of three trials (Cloarec 1992; Pilz 1990; Steiner 1986), which reported adequate data suggested a statistically significant reduction in favour of HCSE compared with placebo (WMD 4.71 mm; 95% CI 1.13 to 8.28; pooled standardised mean difference 0.60; 95% CI 0.15 to 1.05). At the calf, the pooled analysis of three trials (Cloarec 1992; Pilz 1990; Steiner 1986),

25. Significant is often used as a statistical term indicating that the result is unlikely to have occurred by chance.

26. Placebo is a means for differentiating between specific and non-specific effects in clinical trials.

27. Scores can be used to combine data from more than one outcome measure.

28. Scientists usually prefer objective signs to subjective symptoms.

29. A meta-analysis is a method to combine the results of several studies into one overall finding.

30. Confidence intervals are a measure indicating the variation within a set of data.

31. Most trials are superiority trials testing whether one treatment is better than another. Equivalence means not superior but as good (or bad) as the other treatment.

32. The dose is obviously important and can sometimes be used to test for dose-effect relationships.

33. Mean is the sum of all data divided by the number of data.

34. Follow-up describes the length of the observation period.

suggested a statistically significant reduction in favour of HCSE compared with placebo (WMD 3.51 mm; 95% CI 0.58 to 6.45; pooled standardised mean difference 0.42; 95% CI -0.04 to 0.88).

Adverse events

Fourteen studies reported on adverse events.[35] Four studies (Cloarec 1992; Diehm 1996a; Pilz 1990; Rudofsky 1986) reported that there were no treatment-related adverse events in theHCSEgroup. Gastrointestinal complaints, dizziness, nausea, headache and pruritus[36] were reported as adverse events in six studies (Diehm 2000; Friederich 1978; Morales 1993; Neiss 1976; Rehn 1996; Steiner 1990a). The frequency ranged from 1 to 36%[37] of treated patients. Four other studies (Diehm 1992; Koch 2002; Lohr 1986; Steiner 1986) reported good tolerability with HCSE.

Discussion[38]

35. Adverse events are undesirable incidence occurring during the study.

36. It is essential to know what they are…

37. …and how frequently they occur.

38. The discussion follows. It is not reprinted here but can be found in the originally article (www.cochrane.org). The importance of a good discussion was explained previously.

CHAPTER 4 **GETTING INVOLVED IN RESEARCH**

A step by step approach

It is clear that most healthcare practitioners will not get involved in actually doing research – but some might. The following is an attempt to provide a brief outline of how healthcare practitioners might go about planning this. My aim is to save you from at least some of the many mistakes I have committed in my own career. The guide has to be used flexibly: the only golden rule is that there are no golden rules.

Motivations for doing research

Numerous reasons for doing research exist, and some are clearly better than others. Enthusiastic clinicians usually want to prove that 'their' therapy works. Paradoxically, this is one of the worst motivations. An investigation should not set out to prove a point but must test a hypothesis. An investigator with strong preconceptions is hardly an objective researcher, and objectivity is an essential hallmark of all good research.

The type of research in which healthcare practitioners might get involved is clinical research which must be patient centred. The best reason for doing research therefore is the hope to come one step closer to the truth and to improve future healthcare. It is important to realize that both a positive or a negative result will achieve this aim. The most important characteristic of the result, it seems to follow, is not its direction (negative or positive) but its conclusiveness.

There have been as great contributions to improved healthcare through a research programme showing that a long established treatment was not effective as there have been contributions that proved that a new treatment was effective.

When working as a researcher you should only be interested in finding out the truth and then reporting it.

Various preconditions

Certain things are essential preconditions for doing research; without them there is no use even attempting. It is worth remembering that bad research can be (and usually is) unethical – it involves wasting resources and perhaps even needless suffering of patients. Knowledge of research methodology and of the subject area under investigation (e.g. treatment modality and disease) are absolute prerequisites.

Getting expert help

What if, in a given setting, methodological expertise does not exist? To some degree expertise can be 'bought in', but the leader of a research project must have some understanding of all the major issues involved. So, if you do not have this expertise, go and acquire it. If you cannot acquire it or don't want to do so, you should not embark on research in a leading role.

Support services

Infrastructure is also essential. You simply cannot do without things like the time to carry out the work, access to a library, electronic databases and computers, a sufficient number and variety of patients as well as the funds to finance all the activities involved. Draw up a checklist at the outset of your project of all the preconditions required in your particular case and then go through it one by one. Table 1 lists some items that will often prove to be relevant.

Background reading

Let's assume you may want to embark on a study of aromatherapy for asthma. You may not be fully aware of what has been published on this subject. It is mandatory that you catch up and read what others have done before you. It is even advisable to conduct an in-depth search for all published articles, read all of them thoroughly and make sure you understand all aspects of this research – if you do not, you should seek help.

Failure to do this background research thoroughly might embarrass you later on – you might, for instance, find out that the study you have just concluded has already been conducted in a more definitive way by someone else. This would obviously render your

Table 1 – Checklist of items that often are essential preconditions for conducting research

Preconditions
Computers
Dedication
Ethical approval (informed consent)
Expertise (various types, see text)
Funds
Knowledge of previous work in this area
Library access
Measurement devices
Motivation (see text)
Patient access
Space (e.g. clinical laboratory)
Support (e.g. from your superior or organisation)
Time

work more or less redundant. Background reading demands a lot: time, dedication, understanding, library support and other items listed in table 1.

Again: the research question

I keep coming back to this – it shows you how important it is. You may have started out with the idea of studying aromatherapy for asthma. After reading the published articles on the subject, you will probably have found that the question you are asking is much more complex than originally anticipated.

Is your project about formulating or testing a hypothesis? What type of patients do you want to study? What type of aromatherapy using which oils and in what concentrations? How do you want to recruit your clients? How many do you need? Do you need to conduct a **controlled trial** or an **observational study**? What should the control treatment be? Does a good (credible, indistinguishable from the real treatment) 'placebo' (or sham) treatment for aromatherapy exist? Do you need to **randomise** your patients? Can you **blind** the study participants? Is the treatment under investigation representative for its class? How often should patients be treated? Are all conditions optimal for the treatment to work? Do you need one or more therapists? What is the best statistical approach to evaluate your data?

You are likely to find that the list of questions that require answering grows longer by the minute. Only when you have answered all of them will you be able to define the research question adequately. Doing this is essential for deciding which methodology is the best for the project that is evolving in you mind; it is also a decisive step towards developing a **protocol**.

Logistics

This preparatory work will have led you to a more concise idea of what is coming up. You might, at this stage, want to (re)check whether the logistic preconditions for your research project are fulfilled. For instance, do you have access to the type (and adequate numbers) of patients you want to study? Is it realistic for you to obtain the right amount of funding? Is it likely that you can obtain patient consent for what you plan to do? Is the evolving proposal ethical? Do you have the necessary rooms, and manpower (secretarial back-up, research assistants etc)?

There will be many other questions to ask. My advice is again to draw up a checklist and tackle one problem at a time.

Sadly, it is at this stage that many enthusiastically conceived research projects come to a premature end. Many healthcare practitioners who come to my unit for advice on research are overwhelmed with the obstacles that keep emerging and simply give up. But there often is no other choice – research is never easy and there can be no shortcuts to scientific rigour.

The research team

But let's assume you don't give up. By now you will have found that your research knowledge and clinical experience are insufficient to cover all aspects of your project competently. This is no reason for embarrassment; the situation might only get embarrassing if you are not open about your own limitations and pretend to know everything.

This is the time to assemble a team for developing a formal protocol of your study and guide you through its experimental phase. Depending on the type of your project, this team will vary in size. In the above example (aromatherapy for asthma) it might include
1. a statistician,

2. a chest physician and

3. one or more experienced aromatherapists.

Types of research studies

This is a short summary of the sometimes confusing array of terminology applied for different types of studies. More detailed definitions are offered in chapter 5.

Case controlled study: comparison between a group of individuals that have with another that do not have a certain characteristic.

Case series: description of several patients that are of particular interest.

Clinical trial or controlled clinical trial: description of several patients that are of particular interest.

Cohort study: see observational study.

Cross-over trial: a trial where two groups of patients receive two treatments in a different sequence.

Cross sectional study: an investigation of a group of people at one particular point in time.

Equivalence trial: study testing whether two treatments generate similar results.

Individual patient trial: study involving one single patient only.

Mega-trial: study with a particularly large sample size

Meta-analysis: the statistical pooling of data from several single trials to generate a new overall result.

Multi-centre trial: study performed in numerous locations.

Non-experimental study: see observational study.

Observational study: study without a control group where effects of an intervention are observed.

Open-label trial: study without blinding

Pilot study: study to access the feasibility of a protocol.

Post-marketing surveillance study: large observational study for monitoring adverse effects.

Pragmatic trial: study testing the effectiveness of an intervention in a real life situation.

Preclinical study: study with human volunteers under strictly controlled conditions.

Preference trial: study accounting for patients preferences between two or more interventions

Prevention trial: study testing the effectiveness of a preventative measure.

Prospective study: study that records events prospectively.

Retrospective study: study that records events retrospectively.

Single-case study: see individual patient trial.

Superiority trial: study testing whether one treatment is better than another one.

Systematic review: analysis of the totality of the evidence in a transparent, reproducible fashion.

Make the team as small as possible but as large as necessary. You should now organise a series of 'round table' discussions to develop a protocol. Subsequently, you might take the lead and draft a written outline and circulate it within the team until every member of your team is happy with all aspects of the project.

The team should then not disband, but supervise and monitor the entire investigation. Once the protocol is finalised, the planning phase is (almost) finished. All that is needed now is to submit it to the appropriate ethics committee, and secure funding. This may require several, hopefully small, revisions of your protocol.

Funding research

Funding is, of course, very often the stumbling point. More often than not we get rejected with our applications. This always is extremely disappointing. But don't be deterred. To succeed you have to try over and over again. Seek expert advice. Consult your team. Try your local Research and Development Office, establish contact with patient organisations, try all the charities you can think of, use your imagination and leave no stone unturned.

If your project is in the area of CAM, things may be particularly difficult. In the UK, hardly any dedicated funds for CAM research exist. Thus CAM researchers find themselves competing with those from mainstream medicine for a more and more limited budget. This means that our applications are judged by panels who usually have little understanding of and even less sympathy for CAM. Thus the NHS spends only 0.08% and UK medical charities spend 0.05% of their research budgets on CAM research – hardly sums that are in proportions with the increasing usage of CAM by those who gave this money in the first place!

However, CAM has its supporters. The Foundation for Integrated Health is one body that seeks to foster research into CAM treatments and may be able to advise.

Conclusion

Careful planning is essential for any type of research. Omitting this crucial preparatory work is a recipe for failure. But sadly, doing all the necessary planning is not a guarantee for success – it merely renders it more likely.

CHAPTER 5 **IMPORTANT CONCEPTS AND EXPLANATIONS – YOUR ALPHABETICAL GUIDE TO RESEARCH TERMS**

The terminology and 'language' of research

No one involved in reading or using research in any form can do so without understanding the key terms and concepts used in research reports. Researchers have built up a whole 'language' and terminology to enable them to deal precisely with the various aspects of research. The terms have precise definitions, and it is crucial to understand them – if not confusion and misunderstandings are inevitable. Some terms are easier to understand than others. So don't get frustrated if you do not get the meaning of this or that – given time and experience it will all become clear.

As you start reading research reports regularly, you will become familiar with these terms and their meanings, where they are used and how to understand what they are depicting. As you start in research awareness you may need a reference list of all the common terms used.

This section provides an alphabetical list of the most important terms and concepts. Here you will get the full explanation while in earlier section a simplified definition or explanation may have been given to enable you to understand the point being made.

Your reference guide

This is the central part of the book. Its purpose is to serve as a reference: when you read research articles, you come across terms which may be unfamiliar or words that you don't understand. Hopefully you will find them explained in this section. In addition to providing definitions this section aims at explaining important concepts in medical research. It is therefore worth browsing through it and, when needed, referring to it when specific terms require clarification. You are NOT expected to learn them all!

Term	Description	Example of use/Comment
Accuracy	is the proportion of all results, e.g. of a diagnostic test, which are correct.	A test must be accurate in order to be useful.
Active control	Instead of using a placebo, one can use a standard treatment of known and generally accepted efficacy as a comparator in clinical trials. This is called an 'active control'.	A trial of the herbal antidepressant St John's Wort might use a conventional antidepressant drug of known efficacy as a comparator.

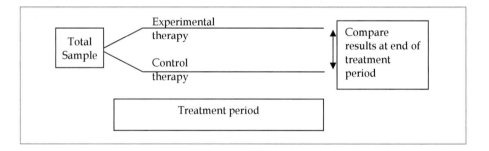

Term	Description	Example of use/Comment
Adherence	See Compliance.	
Adjunctive therapy	Any treatment that is used as an 'add on' to another medical intervention, also called concomitant therapy.	In a study of massage for cancer, all patients would, for obvious reasons, need to receive conventional cancer therapy. Thus massage would be an adjunctive therapy.
Adverse drug reaction (ADR)	Undesirable outcome after taking a medicine. There are, of course, adverse effects after most treatments, not just drugs.	Some patients may experience an allergic reaction after taking a herbal remedy – this would be an ADR.

Term	Description	Example of use/Comment
Adverse effect	Undesirable outcome due to a medical intervention. Often the term **side-effect** is used instead of adverse effect. However, this is not quite correct – an adverse effect is always negative and a side-effect can be positive. For instance, a patient might receive massage therapy for back pain and not that he subsequently sleeps better – this could be a side-effect of the massage.	Some patients feel drowsy after an acupuncture session which might interfere with their ability to drive a car. This would be an adverse effect.
Adverse event	Undesirable incident which may or many not be related to a medical intervention – even if there is no causality, e.g. a patient suffers a stroke while having a course of Bach Flower Remedies, the stroke would still be called an adverse event.	In a clinical trial of therapeutic touch, some patients may fall ill, for instance, from a common cold. This would be an adverse event almost certainly unrelated to therapeutic touch.
Allocation	Any method of assigning patients to treatment groups, e.g. experimental (A) or control group (B), in **clinical trials**.	There are several methods of allocation, e.g. by patient preference or by randomisation.

Term	Description	Example of use/Comment
Allopathy	A term invented by Samuel Hahnemann, the founder of homeopathy, to describe the treatments of mainstream medicine.	The term was meant to be derogatory but has nevertheless become widely used.
Anamnesis	The taking and evaluation of a case history. Different schools of medicine have vastly different ways of taking a medical history.	For instance, a homeopathic anamnesis is dramatically different from a conventional medical history.
Antagonist	An agent that opposes, impedes or neutralises the action of another agent.	The term is used for chemical substance in science and for people in everyday language.

Term	Description	Example of use/Comment
Artefact	A result which was not caused by the factor under investigation but by another circumstance.	If, for instance, a form of electrotherapy does not generate any benefit, this could simply be due to the fact that the machine was not switched on.
Association	Describes the occurrence of two events together; an association may or may not be causal.	For instance, teenage sex and teenage pregnancy are causally associated but the number of storks and the birth rate are not – even if they should occur together.
Attrition	Is the loss of patients included in a clinical trial; it can be due to a range of factors which may or may not be related to the study.	For instance, a patient moving home would be unrelated, and patient experiencing adverse effects would be related to the investigation.
Audit	Is a set of principles originating from the world of finance which are now applied also to medicine. It describes an official examination of accounts. In medicine, it is often wrongly seen as a form of research. Audit is audit and not research! Typically an audit follows a cyclical pattern asking a sequence of questions: 1. Where are we? 2. Where do we want to be? 3. How do we get there?	An audit of an acupuncture practice might help to treat more patients more efficiently. An audit of hospital hygiene might identify deficiencies and ways to remedy them.
Autonomy	Is each individual's capacity and right for self-determination. In medical research, autonomy determines a person's right to say no, i.e. to refuse to participate or co-operate.	In medical ethics, autonomy is a fundamental principle guaranteeing patient's rights.
Autoregulation	Mechanisms by which the body is able to self-regulate functions or adapt to new situations.	For instance, if we live at high altitude for a long period of time, our physiology adapts in numerous ways to circumstances such as low oxygen concentration of the air.

Term	Description	Example of use/Comment
Baseline characteristics	In **longitudinal studies** or **clinical trials**, patients can be characterised by a set of variables including age, sex, body weight etc at entry; these are called baseline characteristics (or data).	Baseline characteristics are important in several ways. For instance, if other researchers wanted to replicate the study they would need to recruit patients that have a similar profile.
Basement-effect	If, in a **clinical trial**, values are already fairly low to start with, it is difficult for any intervention to lower them further. (See also **ceiling effect**.)	For example, a clinical trial of acupuncture for pain control is bound to show no effect if most of the included patients only had little or no pain.
Basic research	A term used for non-clinical research.	For instance, test-tube experiments to identify the mechanisms of action of a treatment or the mechanisms involved in disease. The opposite of basic research is applied (or, in medicine, clinical) research.
Before-after analysis (or comparison)	In **observational studies**, measurements are usually taken at the outset of, during and after an intervention. Subsequently, these measurements are compared to each other generating the perceived therapeutic effect (PTE)	It is tempting but wrong to think of the PTE as being the singular result of the treatment. In fact, the PTE may be caused by a range of factors including: · **natural history** of the condition (most diseases get better without any therapy) · **regression towards the mean** (extreme values tend to return towards the average) · **social desirability** (many patients tend to exaggerate benefits in an attempt to please the therapist) · concomitant treatments (many patients use other treatments simultaneously which they don't tell us about, **adjunctive treatments**) In **controlled clinical trials**, one therefore compares two groups of patients which have all or most of these factors in common and only differ in terms of the treatment that is being tested. In this case, any difference should be due to that intervention.

See table overleaf...

Term	Description	Example of use/Comment

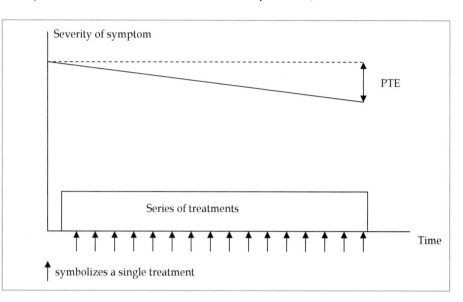

Beneficence	The principle of doing good is a cornerstone of medical ethics. It must not be violated or else the research is likely to be unethical.	The determination to do the best for their patients is something that clinicians of all types have in common.
Benefit	In medical terms, 'benefit' is used to describe the fact that a treatment promotes or enhances well-being or produces a (health) advantage.	When talking about benefit, it is crucial to define the perspective. The patient's perspective, for instance, could be different from that of society at large.
Best-case series	Is a series of cases which all suggest a positive outcome after an intervention. Best-case series can generate **hypotheses** but cannot test them.	For instance, a series of cancer patients may have all responded well to treatment with the herbal mixture Essiac. This would then encourage other researchers to design a clinical trial testing its efficacy.
Best evidence synthesis	A form of **systematic review** that tries to account for the quality of the evidence. In essence, the totality of the available evidence is evaluated but the conclusions are based mainly on the data that are the most reliable.	As poor quality studies can generate misleading results, it is crucial to take account of a quality when evaluating published studies.

Term	Description	Example of use/Comment
Bias	Is any systematic deviation of the truth. Bias therefore renders the results of research unreliable. Rigorous research aims at minimizing bias.	There are numerous sources of bias including · **Attrition bias**: occurs when many patients are lost in a clinical trial but are not properly accounted for in the analysis. For instance, a certain treatment may cause severe **adverse effects** in some patients prompting them to leave the trial. If these cases are simply not analysed, a misleadingly positive result may occur. · **Financial support bias**: commercially sponsored research often turns out to be more positive than research not supported in that way. · **Journal bias**: some journal editors seem to have strong preferences. For instance, the most prestigious of all medical journal 'The New England Journal of Medicine' has, to the best of my knowledge, never published a single positive study of CAM – but numerous negative articles on CAM have appeared in that journal. · **Language bias**: we know that Chinese studies tend to report positive results. In fact, according to one survey, there is not a single negative trial of acupuncture that originates from China! A review of these studies would therefore invariably generate positive evidence which may be misleading. · **'Not my scene' bias**: occurs when people belittle the importance of a subject area. For instance, there is evidence that reviewers are, on average, more critical of a trial of homeopathy compared to an otherwise identical study of a conventional drug.

Term	Description	Example of use/Comment
		· **Publication bias**: positive results tend to get published, while many negative findings remain unpublished. This phenomenon therefore distorts the evidence of **systematic reviews**. · **Selection bias**: imaging a controlled clinical trial where patients were allowed to select to have acupuncture or placebo treatment for their pain. Those who selected acupuncture would tend to expect a good result from it. This expectation can produce a positive outcome unrelated to the effects of acupuncture. The best way to minimize selection bias is **randomisation**.
Biological plausibility	The degree to which the assertion of a **cause-effect relationship** is consistent with our knowledge of the mechanisms of disease.	Many CAM interventions (e.g. homeopathy or therapeutic touch) have a low level of biological plausibility.
Black box approach	To test the value of **complex interventions** which consist of several treatments, one could either test each of them separately (**reductionism**) or one could test them when they are applied together. The latter option is the black box approach.	For instance, if we needed to know whether classical homeopathy, which is highly individualised, is effective, one could test whether patients consulting a classical homeopath fare better than those who don't. This test would be regardless of the remedies that are being prescribed by the therapist. In fact, it might include dozens of different remedies. It therefore does not test a single remedy but treats homeopathy as a 'black box' and test it in its entirety.
Blinding	Is the method of concealment in a clinical trial.	If trial participants, e.g. patients or therapists, are not blinded to treatment allocation, they might have certain expectations which impact on the results. The parties that can be blinded are

Term	Description	Example of use/Comment
		• the patients • the therapist • the nurse making the outcome measurements • the statistician doing the analyses
Bonferroni adjustment	Statistical adjustment for conducting multiple tests of probability.	For instance, if one performs 20 different tests at the 5% level of **statistical, significance**, one would generate a positive result purely by chance. To avoid this error one can use **Bonferroni's method**.
Carry-over effects	Effects of a medical intervention which are long-lasting and could therefore affect the results of a **cross-over trial**. Because in a cross-over trial, all patients receive a succession of two or more treatments, prolonged effects from treatment phase 1 could impact on the outcome in phase 2.	For instance, a cross-over study of acupuncture might mean that some patients are first treated for 4 weeks and then observed for 4 weeks without receiving acupuncture. If acupuncture has long-lasting effects, these carry-over effects would influence the results in the second four weeks.
Case-control study	An **observational study** in which the 'cases' but not the 'controls' are exposed to the factor or characteristic under investigation.	Typical examples include comparisons of • smokers with non-smokers • stroke patients with individuals without a stroke (or any other condition) • people who use CAM with people who don't use it • people who have pets with those who don't have pets • workers who have been exposed to asbestos with those who haven't • women who had children with those who didn't Case-control studies are often relatively easy and inexpensive to perform and can shed some light on unexpected events. They cannot, however, prove the existence of a **causal relationship**.

Term	Description	Example of use/Comment
Case report	This term is a description of the circumstances of a particularly noteworthy patient or case.	For instance, in terms of a remarkably **positive outcome** or of an important **adverse event**.
Case series	If more than one patient is being described in this way, we speak of a case-series.	A case series could, for instance, describe 10 patients with depression who all improved after receiving regular treatments with stroking back massages.
Causal relationship or cause-effect relationship	An association where one circumstance or event brings about another.	For instance, smoking causes lung cancer. Causality can sometimes be wrongly assumed and must therefore always be proven rather than assumed. An **association** of two events does not prove causality. For instance, long-term cigarette smoking also causes yellow discolouring of the 2nd and 3rd fingers. Someone might have observed that yellow fingers and lung cancer are associated and wrongly concluded that there is a causal relationship between the two. Establishing causality is crucial for effective interventions: bleaching yellow fingers does not prevent lung cancer but smoking cessation does!
Cause	A circumstance or factor that directly brings about change.	The cause of pregnancy is sexual intercourse. One cause of lung cancer can be smoking.
Ceiling effect	If the **primary outcome measure** in a clinical trial is not very pathological to start with, there may not be any room for significant improvement. This phenomenon it called the ceiling effect.	Imagine, for instance, a study with back pain patients where it turns out that many patients had, in fact, very high mobility to start with. Then there is no room for improvement of this outcome measure. Ceiling effects may contribute to **type II errors** or **false negative results**. (See also **basement effect**.)

Term	Description	Example of use/Comment
Chance	The cause of random variation.	Chance can play 'dirty tricks' in research and rigorous research designs have the aim to limit the impact of chance on the result.
Clinical significance (or relevance)	If the results of a **clinical trial** are not due to **chance**, they are **statistically significant**. Many observers have commented that too much emphasis is put on this type of significance in medical research. A finding may be statistically significant and, at the same time, clinically meaningless, i.e. devoid of clinical relevance.	For instance, a **meta-analysis** of clinical trials of garlic supplements may show that it lowers blood pressure in a statistically significant way. The reduction is, however, so small that it is meaningless and thus not clinically significant or relevant. There are no definitive rules as to what is and what is not clinically significant. A 2% reduction of blood pressure is probably not clinically relevant, while a 2% reduction of mortality may well be. The decision essentially amounts to a clinical judgment. It is advisable to define at the outset of a clinical trial what the investigators regard as clinically significant.
Clinical trial or controlled clinical trial	An experiment where one group of patients is treated for the purpose of that investigation with an '**experimental**' (or **verum**) treatment, i.e. the therapy that is being tested, and another group receives another treatment, i.e. the control or **comparison group**.	The control group might receive any of the following interventions: · no treatment at all · treatment as usual · a gold standard treatment or **active control** · a **placebo**

Clinical trials can have various aims:

1. Most frequently they test the **efficacy** or **effectiveness** of treatments.
2. They can also test the effectiveness/efficacy of preventative measures.
3. They can test the best ways of diagnosing diseases and health problems.

Term	Description	Example of use/Comment
Cochrane Collaboration	International network of people who conduct independent **systematic reviews** usually of high quality which are subsequently published on the Cochrane Database (**www.thecochranelibrary.com**).	These reviews are generally considered to provide the most reliable information available covering all areas of healthcare. Cochrane groups exist in all areas of medicine, also in CAM.
Cohort-study	An **observational study** of a particular group of people or patients over time.	For instance, if we monitor the next 100 patients who receive acupuncture for pain control, this would be a cohort study.
Comparison group	The group of patients in a clinical trail that does not receive the **experimental treatment** but a **control intervention control group**.	The comparison group could receive: 1. no treatment at all, 2. another treatment, 3. a placebo or sham treatment.
Complex interventions	Treatments which consist of more than one component that act both independently and interdependently.	It could be argued, for instance, that homeopathy is a complex intervention consisting of 1) the remedy, 2) the typical history taking and 3) the therapist patient interaction. It could also be argued that most medical treatments are complex.
Compliance or adherence	A measure of the extent to which patients follow advice in clinical practice or a protocol in medical research.	For instance, one may read that '80% of patients were fully compliant with the treatment'. Essentially this means that 80% administered the therapy as advised. It is essential to monitor compliance. Patients may, for instance, not take a herbal remedy because it tastes awful. If the researchers were unaware of this lack of compliance they might wrongly conclude that the remedy did not work.
Confidence interval	A statistical measure of the degree of uncertainty associated with a given result. It signifies the range of numbers within which the true result lies.	Aromatherapy, for instance, might be shown to reduce stress in 8 patients by 10% on average of 10%. This result could have been generated by two dramatically different scenarios. In scenario [A], all patients benefit in a similar fashion; in scenario [B] only few patients do.

Term	Description	Example of use/Comment

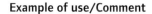

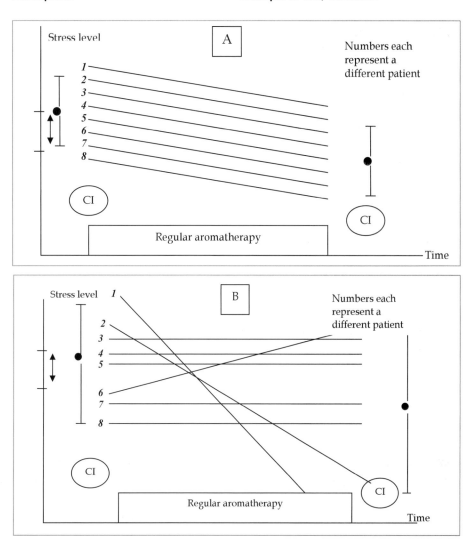

The upper and lower limits of the confidence intervals (CI) tell us that, in [A], we can be relatively certain about the effect while, in [B], we cannot. Conventionally, confidence intervals are expressed as '95% confidence intervals', often abbreviated as '95% CI'. This means that 95% of all the individual data lie in the range provided. Confidence intervals can be expressed graphically as in the above figures or numerically, e.g. 95% CI = 1.3-10.8.

Term	Description	Example of use/Comment
Confidentiality	Even though researchers should publish their results, the data of individual study participants are always confidential. Breach of patient confidentiality would be unethical. It is only allowed with written agreement.	Confidentiality is an important ethical principle to which all clinicians are bound. Violation of confidentiality may result in disciplinary action.

Term	Description	Example of use/Comment
Conflict of interest	This is a self-explanatory term. Usually conflicts of interest focus on financial support and sponsorship. However, there are other conceivable conflicts.	For instance, Reiki healers may conduct a clinical trial without outside financial support but they may have strong conviction about the value of Reiki. This may present an important conflict of interest for conducting unbiased research in this area.
Confounders	These are factors, other that the one under investigation, that influence the outcome.	For instance, in a clinical trial of Reiki for pain, some patients may have taken aspirin which then would be a confounder in that study. Rigorous trial design aims at controlling for confounders. For instance, if in the example of the Reiki trial, patients need to take pain killers, one could make sure that this happens in the control group to the same extent. In this case the influence of this factor on **inter-group differences** would be minimized.
Consent forms	This is a form research subjects sign after being fully informed, to indicate their **informed consent** in participating in the project.	It should tell the patients in understandable language about the purpose and the risks of a study.
Consistency	Constancy of findings when studies are repeated or different types of investigations lead to similar conclusions.	For instance, as all types of studies demonstrate a link between smoking and lung cancer, the finding is likely to be real.
Context-effects	See **Non-specific effects**.	
Continuous variable	Some outcome measurements in **quantitative research** are discrete or categorical (e.g. patient is dead or alive), others are continuous.	Blood pressure, body weight and pain are examples of continuous variables – they can increase or decrease continuously.
Control group	This is the group of patients that is used as a reference or **comparison group** in a clinical trial.	Controls can receive either no treatment at all, an active treatment or a placebo. The results of the control group are compared

Term	Description	Example of use/Comment
		to those in the **experimental group** and are an indicator for the effect caused by the **experimental treatment** or **verum**.
Controlled trial	See **Clinical trial**.	
Correlation	A measure of the **association** between two factors.	The factors may [A] or may not [B] signify a **causal relationship**. [A] and [B] are positive correlations: as one factor increases, the other also increases. [C] shows a negative correlation: as one factor increases, the other decreases.

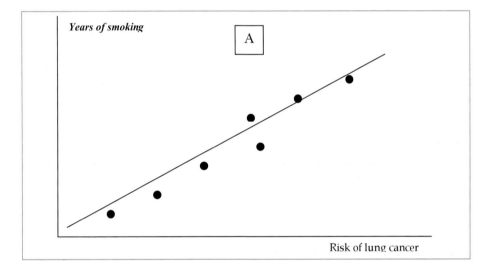

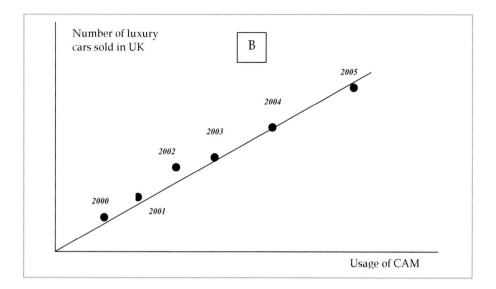

Number of luxury cars sold in UK

B

Usage of CAM

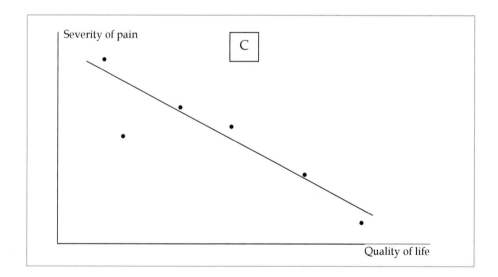

Severity of pain

C

Quality of life

Term	Description	Example of use/Comment
Critical appraisal	Techniques used to scrutinize evidence systematically, consciously and explicitly (see the first section of this book).	Critical appraisal is an important method to identify the strengths and weaknesses of research reports.
Cross-over-trial	A **clinical trial** where patients switch from the **experimental treatment** to the **control intervention**.	Instead of comparing one group of patients with another, the same patients can be compared during exposure to two different interventions.

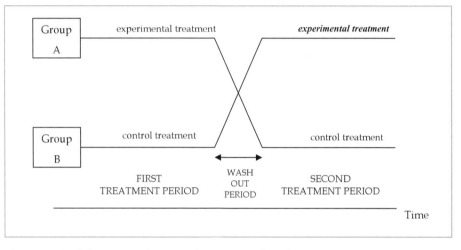

The strength of this approach is that the number of **confounders** can be minimised – each patient is compared with him- or herself. The disadvantages are that such trials are sensitive to other factors such as **carry-over effects**, and that statistical analysis of the results can be complex.

Term	Description	Example of use/Comment
Cross-sectional study	This is an investigation of a group of patients at one particular time point only.	For instance, a study might determine how many hospital patients currently use CAM. Such studies have many limitations, e.g. little ability to demonstrate **causal relationships**, but they certainly can generate interesting **research questions** and are usually quick and relatively inexpensive.

Term	Description	Example of use/Comment
Data dredging	If a set of data is analysed over and over again under different aspects or with different methods until eventually a significant result pops up, this is called **data dredging** (or fishing or mining). The likelihood of **false positive results** increases with the number of analyses.	The proper way to go about data analyses is to predefine in the protocol what the primary analysis will be. If further analyses are desirable, it is important to label them clearly as **exploratory analyses**. These 'post hoc analyses' can be valuable, particularly for generating new **hypotheses** – but they cannot test hypotheses.
Declaration of Helsinki	A set of ethical guidelines set by the World Médical Association (**www.wma.net**) for conducting biomedical research. The first version was adopted in 1964. Since then numerous updates have been issued.	These guidelines are binding for all who conduct medical research.
Dichotomous variable	Variables which can only have two values, e.g. male or female, dead or alive.	Another name for it is categorical. (See also **continuous variable**).
Dose	The amount of a medicine administered to a patient or person.	Usually a very small dose generates no effect and an excessively high dose is toxic.
Dose response (or dose effect)	This is the change in outcome that results from a change in therapeutic dose.	Normally one expects the effect to get larger in proportion with increasing dose – but this is not always the case.

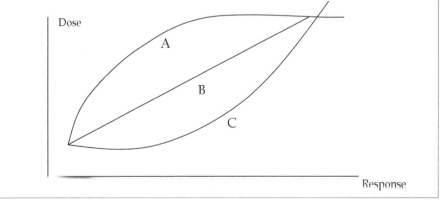

Three different dose response curves A, B, C – all have in common that the response increases as the dose increases. Interestingly, in homeopathy this is assumed to be the reverse: the higher the dilution, the stronger the response – this is one of the reasons why homeopathy is considered implausible by many scientists **biological plausibility**.

Double-blind	A term used for **clinical trials** indicating that the two main parties, i.e. the patient and the clinician, are unaware which treatment is given to which patient.	The aim of blinding is to minimize the influence of expectation on the outcome.
Dropout	If a patient leaves a clinical trial without permission, this is called a dropout.	If a patient leaves with permission, this is called a **withdrawal**. In order to generate reliable results, it is important to account for both dropouts and withdrawals (**attrition bias**).
Economic analysis	This is an analysis of the monetary implications of interventions.	Several types exist: · **Cost-minimisation analysis**: assumes that the outcomes of the two treatments which are being compared are the same – so only their costs differ. · **Cost-effectiveness analysis**: assumes outcomes are not the same and are measured in natural units, e.g. blood pressure. · **Cost-benefit analysis**: outcomes are not the same and measured in monetary units. · **Cost-utility analysis**: outcomes are not the same and measured in terms of utility.
Effect	Is the consequence or result of an intervention or circumstance.	The effect of too much calorie input is obesity. Obesity is the result of too much calorie input.
Effect size	An effect can be anything from tiny to huge. To compare the results of different interventions, one might consider the effect size.	Garlic, for instance, lowers cholesterol levels significantly. Unfortunately, the effect size is considerably smaller than that of conventional lipid-lowering drugs.

Term	Description	Example of use/Comment
Effectiveness	Addresses the question whether a treatment works under real life conditions.	It is conceivable that a given therapy works only under optimal conditions but not in every day practice. For instance, in clinical practice patients may not **comply** with a therapy because it causes **adverse effects**.
Efficacy	Addresses the question whether a treatment works under highly controlled, ideal conditions.	Efficacy studies ask the question, can this treatment work in optimal circumstances?
Eligibility criteria	See **Inclusion criteria/exclusion criteria** and **Entry criteria**.	
Endpoint	This is another term for an outcome measure, often reserved for a **primary outcome measure** of a clinical trial, i.e. the endpoint which has been predefined as the one of primary interest to the study.	A clinical trial might, for instance, determine the effects of massage therapy on the well-being of cancer patients as the primary endpoint. Other (**secondary endpoints**) could be the need for drugs, the cost or rate of adverse effects.
Entry criteria	Are those predefined characteristics or factors which allow a trial participant to become part of a particular study.	For instance, if a new treatment for hypertension is being tested, a main entry criterion might be that each patient has elevated blood pressure.
Equipose	Is a group's position of uncertainty about the value of a treatment.	To conduct a trial of homeopathy versus placebo, for instance, the group of trialists should, as a whole, feel uncertain about the value of homeopathy. If certainty existed, it could be unethical to conduct the trial because then the researchers would feel certain that they deprive those patients who receive placebo of an effective treatment. In such a case, a clinical trial with an **active control** might be the way forward.

Term	Description	Example of use/Comment
Equivalence trial (or non-inferiority trial)	Most trials test whether one treatment is better than another one, for instance, a placebo. The equivalence trial is specifically designed to test whether two therapies have the same or similar effects.	This approach avoids treating one group with a placebo which might be ethically problematic. The disadvantage is that the required sample sizes are usually substantially larger than with **superiority trials**.
Ethics	Medical ethics are a developing set of rules that govern medicine as a whole, including medical research. The four cornerstones of medical ethics are: • beneficence – the determination to do good • non-malevolence– the determination to inflict no harm • autonomy– respect for the self-determination of the individual • justice – determination to be just and fair	Ethics committees or ethical review boards, as they are called in the US, have the task to scrutinise all research projects and make sure they do not violate currently accepted standards. In particular they make sure that: • the potential benefits are greater than the potential for harm to study participants • the information provided to study participants is understandable and complete • the **recruitment procedures** are appropriate • there will is insurance cover in case anything goes wrong Research projects that involve patients or volunteers or animals usually require approval from an ethics committee before they can go ahead.
Evidence-based medicine	This is the systematic, explicit, conscientious and judicious use of evidence when making healthcare decisions.	Recently evidence-based medicine was voted by medical based experts to be among the 15 most important medical innovations of the last two centuries. The principles of evidence-based medicine are applicable to all types of medicine, including CAM (see also other sections of this book).
Exclusion criteria	A set of predefined criteria which prevent a person from participating in a research project.	For instance, a new drug might not be safe for pregnant women. Pregnancy would then be an exclusion criterion. Or a new drug might increase blood pressure – in which case, patients with hypertension should be excluded from a clinical trial of that drug.

Term	Description	Example of use/Comment
Experimental group	The group of patients in a clinical trial that receives the treatment which is being tested. Other names frequently used for the same thing are **intervention group**, **trial group** or **verum group**.	A trial of acupuncture might mean that the experimental group receives acupuncture while the control group receives conventional care.
Experimental treatment	Therapy received by the experimental group, also called **verum group**.	For instance, in a trial of acupuncture versus sham acupuncture, the real acupuncture would be the experimental treatment.
Experimenter effect	According to one theory, the investigator of an experiment influences the result merely by his/her presence.	There is no evidence that experimenter effects exist in rigorous medical research.
Exploratory trial	A trial which is designed not for testing whether a treatment works but for explaining how it works.	If we wanted to find out, for instance, whether homeopathic treatments help patients through the therapeutic encounter with a homeopath, we would need to design an exploratory study to find out.
Exploratory analysis	A **post hoc** analysis of data in order to generate new hypotheses (**data dredging**).	A study of therapeutic touch for eczema might have failed to show significant effects on skin lesions. Yet the researchers might do several exploratory analyses to see whether other variables, e.g. well-being, were affected.
External validity	Describes the extent to which the results of a trial are **generalisable** to other situations.	**Effectiveness trials** often have high external validity. **Efficacy** trials often have low external validity. But this is not an 'either or'; rather it is a continuum or sliding scale.
Factorial design	This is a trial design where two treatments are compared to each other, in combination and to a control.	Schematically, this can be depicted as on the following page:

Term	Description	Example of use/Comment

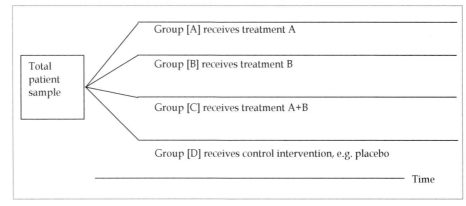

Feasibility trial (or pilot study)

This is a trial which aims to determine the feasibility of a definitive trial to be carried out at a later stage. It aims at answering questions such as:
· Is it possible to recruit enough patients?
· Are all the procedures practical?
· Is the study acceptable to patients?

It is misleading to call a study which turns out to be seriously flawed a pilot study in order to get it published despite its flaws. Such a trial simply is a flawed study.

Focus group

A method frequently used in qualitative research where a group of interacting people are interviewed about their views on a certain subject. Focus groups are an adequate method for generating but not for testing hypotheses.

Focus groups can, for instance, generate hypotheses. Frequently their findings are of debatable generalisability. Focus groups are popular in market research.

Follow-up

The length of time during which patients are observed in **prospective studies** and certain **outcome measures** are recorded.

If the follow-up is too short, effects that do exist may be missed (See also **false negative**).

Funnel plot

This a method of detecting **publication bias**, e.g. the phenomenon that some trials (for instance, those with a negative result) remain unpublished. The **sample size** of single studies is plotted against their **effect size**. This normally generates a symmetrical, funnel-like image [A].

If there is publication bias, gaps in the funnel occur as in [B] and the symmetry of the image is lost.

See tables overleaf…

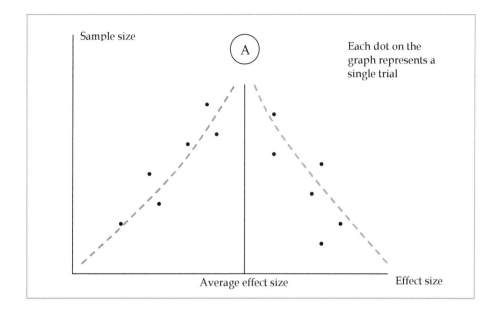

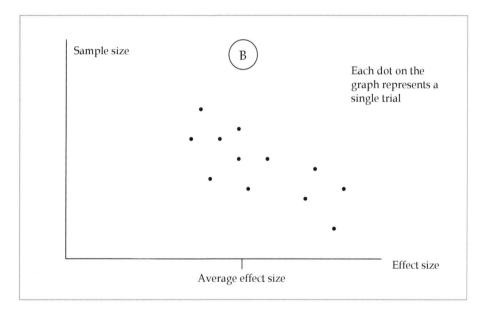

Term	Description	Example of use/Comment
Gold standard	A method that is generally accepted as being the best for a particular purpose.	The gold standard for testing the efficacy of a medical intervention is the randomised clinical trial.
Good clinical practice (GCP)	A set of standards which is continuously being developed and aimed at identifying and promoting high quality in clinical practice.	GCP is important for clinicians of all types. Its aim is to optimise patient-care.
Grey literature	This is a term used to describe publications which are not readily available, e.g. not listed in the commonly used databases such as Medline or Embase. The grey literature usually has to be accessed by hand searching journals and other documents.	If we are interested in Chinese herbal medicine, for instance, the usual databases will contain only a fraction of the published evidence. It can de difficult and time-consuming to access the grey literature – but it can nevertheless be important.
Guidelines	A set of statements aimed at facilitating decision making on a specific subject.	e.g. guidelines for treating back pain effectively.
Hawthorne effect	Those who know that they are part of an experiment can behave differently from normal. When researchers studied the effect of different lighting on productivity in the Hawthorne factory, USA, they found that productivity improved simply because workers were under observation. This can also happen in clinical trials and is a phenomenon which is distinct from the **placebo-effect**.	Placebo, Hawthorne and other effects are usually summarized as **non-specific effects** to distinguish them from the **specific effects** which are directly caused by the treatment.
Health service research	Explores the utility and impact of medical interventions in real life settings.	For instance, evaluating the effects of training nurses in the principles of **evidence-based medicine**.

Term	Description	Example of use/Comment
Heterogeneity	This term indicates difference.	Two or more clinical trials of the same therapy can be different for a vast number of reasons. Imagine, for instance, a trial of acupuncture as a treatment of low back pain. Heterogeneity may occur for a range of reasons, e.g.: · Different types of acupuncture were used (e.g. needle or electro-acupuncture). · Different treatment schedules may have been applied (e.g. 3 x per week or only one single session). · Different patients may have been enrolled (e.g. acute or chronic pain). · Different settings (e.g. secondary or primary care environment). · Different **outcome measures** (pain or mobility).
Hierarchy of evidence	Some types of evidence are more reliable or conclusive than others. Opinion, for instance, counts less than the results of a proper study. This phenomenon can be expressed as a hierarchy. Several slightly different hierarchies have been proposed. At the lower end of the hierarchy is expert opinion; somewhere in the middle are single clinical trials at the top of the hierarchy usually is a **systematic review** of the totality of the available evidence.	The graph below schematically depicts this situation.

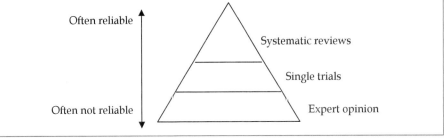

Term	Description	Example of use/Comment
Historical controls	Are patients from the past who have not been exposed to the treatment under investigation.	For instance, when a new therapy has been developed, it may be prudent to first test it on a few volunteers and compare the results to similar cases from the past which did not have that treatment. This can be a good starting point for further research, e.g. it can help generate a hypothesis . However, rarely does it generate conclusive results and it often overestimates the effect size of the new therapy. Thus it is not an adequate design feature for studies aimed at testing hypotheses.
Holism	The concept of viewing patients or systems as a whole, i.e. as more than the sum of their organs or parts.	The concept of holism is fundamental to all good medicine, not just to CAM. (See also **reductionism**).
Hypothesis	A statement or assumption which can be scientifically tested.	This is a different way of approaching the issue of a research question: · **Research question**: is acupuncture effective for acute back pain compared to placebo? · **Hypothesis**: acupuncture is effective for acute back pain compared to placebo · **Null-hypothesis**: acupuncture is not more effective for acute back pain compared to placebo
Iatrogenic effects	Are effects that are caused by a medical intervention, e.g. **adverse-effects** or **side-effects**.	Iatrogenic effects sadly are the cause of much illness and collectively lead to enormous costs.
Incidence	Number of new cases that occur in a given time period.	Incidence = number of new cases in a time period divided by the number of individuals exposed to the risk during that period x 1000. For instance, if in a given time 5 strokes occurred in 10,000 patients receiving spinal manipulation, the incidence (1) would be Incidence = $5 \div 10,000 \times 1000 = 0.5$.

Term	Description	Example of use/Comment
Inclusion criteria	See **Entry criteria**.	
Independent replication	An important principle in science; the results of one single experiment or study can be wrong for many reasons. If we have two or more similar results, we can be more confident. And if we have confirmation from other researchers, we can be even more confident that our results are true.	Few people would accept a new drug purely on the evidence provided by the manufacturer. If an independent group, however, confirms the manufacturer's findings, chances for acceptance increase.
Indiosyncratic	Abnormal and rare, i.e. uncommon reaction after a medical intervention.	Most ingested substances can cause allergies in some people: an idiosyncratic reaction.
Individual patient trial, or n=1, or n of 1 trial	This is a trial with only one patient.	For instance, one individual can be treated in random sequence by either an experimental treatment or a placebo. This would be a randomized, placebo-controlled, double-blind n of one trial. The figure schematically depicts a n=1 trial.

N=1 trials generate valuable information about one patient, e.g. it can answer the questions, does he or she respond to the experimental therapy? They do however, not normally provide data which are generalisable to other patients.

Term	Description	Example of use/Comment
Inference	The process of drawing conclusions from observing a relatively small number of observations about all such cases.	For instance, if we conduct a survey in Devon on 100 back pain patients and find that 90% had tried CAM for treating their problem, we might infer that 90% of all UK back pain patients use CAM. The example shows how careful one has to be about making inference: the population of Devon almost certainly is not representative of the UK population at large.
Informed consent	Voluntary agreement of a person to participate in research or to be given a treatment. The information provided has to be complete, particularly in relation to the risks that the treatment may cause. It also has to be understandable. For research purposes the consent should be given in writing. Failing to obtain informed consent violates ethical, moral and legal rules.	In exceptional circumstances, e.g. research with people who are not mentally competent (e.g. patients suffering from advanced Alzheimer's disease) or investigations on young children, individuals can be entered into a research project without their own consent. In these cases, the next of kin or parents/ guardians usually have to provide informed consent for them.
Intention to treat analysis	Is an analysis of trial data that includes all patients initially entered in the study – even those who **dropped out** or were **withdrawn**.	If data for these patients are not available, strategies exist to create missing values based on certain assumptions. Intention to treat analyses are important for generating reliable information about the **effectiveness** of a therapy. Imagine, for instance, a treatment which has **adverse effects** that are unacceptable to a large proportion of patients. These patients are likely to **drop out**. An intention to treat analysis would correctly show that the therapy is not effective, while a '**per protocol' analysis** might wrongly suggest that it is. This example illustrates that a treatment can be efficacious without being effective.

Term	Description	Example of use/Comment
Inter-group difference	The difference in outcome between two groups of a clinical trial.	Controlled clinical trials have the purpose of generating inter-group differences not **intra-group** (or within group) differences.

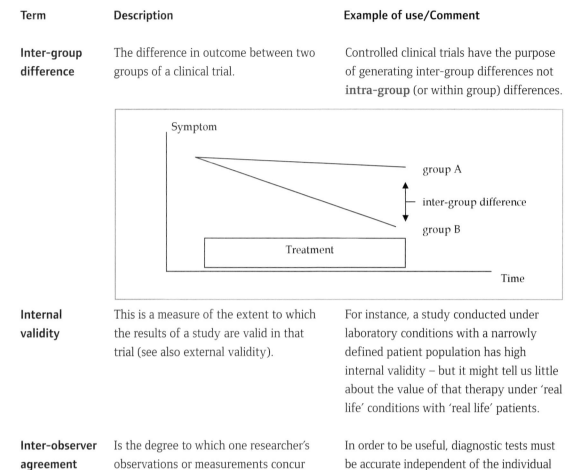

Term	Description	Example of use/Comment
Internal validity	This is a measure of the extent to which the results of a study are valid in that trial (see also external validity).	For instance, a study conducted under laboratory conditions with a narrowly defined patient population has high internal validity – but it might tell us little about the value of that therapy under 'real life' conditions with 'real life' patients.
Inter-observer agreement	Is the degree to which one researcher's observations or measurements concur with those of another.	In order to be useful, diagnostic tests must be accurate independent of the individual who uses them. If applied kinesiology, for instance, fails to have a good inter-observer agreement, its **validity** is debatable.
Intra-group difference	If, in a clinical study, we compare the before-after difference in outcome within one group, this generates the intra-group difference.	**Controlled clinical trials** are for comparing two groups. To rely solely on intra-group differences in such a trial is not correct.

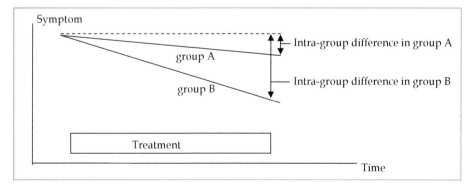

Term	Description	Example of use/Comment
Levels of evidence	See **Hierarchy of evidence**.	
Life table analysis	Analysis, usually graphical, of probability of an event, e.g. death, versus time.	The graphical depiction of a life table analysis reveals more than the end result; It also shows the speed by which an effect occurs.

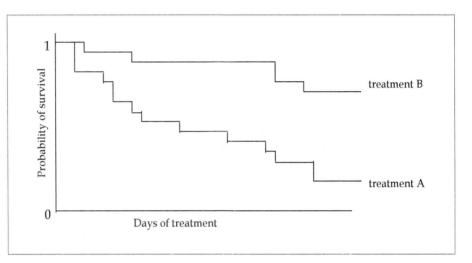

Term	Description	Example of use/Comment
Longitudinal study	Any study which observes patients during a period of time, e.g. by making repeated measurements.	The opposite is a **cross-sectional study**.
Masking	See **Blinding**.	
Matched pair comparison	Instead of **randomizing patients** to two treatments A or B in a **controlled clinical trial**, one could match them such that important characteristics (e.g. gender, body weight, severity of symptom, length of history) are the same in both groups.	This method has the disadvantage that one can never match for characteristics which are not known at the time – and it would be naïve to assume we already know all characteristics which influence any given outcome.

Term	Description	Example of use/Comment
Mean	The sum of observations divided by the number of observations **normal distribution**.	The mean is frequently used to express data of more than one case.

$$\left.\begin{matrix}1\\2\\3\\4\end{matrix}\right\} \text{mean} = 10:4 = 2.5 \qquad \left.\begin{matrix}1\\2\\3\\10\end{matrix}\right\} \text{mean} = 16:4 = 4$$

$$\left.\begin{matrix}1\\2\\3\\4\end{matrix}\right\} \text{median} - 2.5 \qquad \left.\begin{matrix}1\\2\\3\\10\end{matrix}\right\} \text{median} = 2.5$$

Term	Description	Example of use/Comment
Median	The point where the number of observations above equals the number of observations below that point.	Median and mean are rarely the same, depending on the distribution of the data. (See also **normal distribution**.)
Medline	Most frequently used electronic database for medical articles.	Medline can be accessed on **www.ncbi.nlm.nih.gov/entrez**
Mega-trial	This is a trial with a very large **sample size**.	Such trials usually are **multicentre trials** and often have a fairly simple design.
Meta-analysis	This is a form of **systematic review** which includes statistical pooling of the data from several studies thus generating a new 'overall' result. In order to pool data in this way, certain conditions have to be met. For instance, there must not be a high degree of **heterogeneity** between single studies.	If multiple studies exist for therapeutic touch, but their results are not uniform, one might be able to create a conclusive answer by pooling the data of all these trials.
Morbidity	A term to reflect a state of health.	The morbidity in older populations for instance, is generally higher than that of younger ones – which means older people are more frequently ill.
Mortality	A term to signify death	Mortality is always 100% – we all have to die. Healthcare can merely try to delay death and make the quality of life until death better.

Term	Description	Example of use/Comment
Multicentre trial	Is a study which is carried out in more than one location.	This offers the advantage of relatively quickly recruiting larger number of patients. The disadvantage may be that different centres perform differently thus creating a degree of **heterogeneity**.
Multiple outcome measures	The use of more than one outcome measure in a piece of research.	If many endpoints are evaluated in a research project, one might come up **significant results** purely by chance; it is therefore important to control for this factor which is possible through relatively simple statistics (See also **Bonferroni adjustment**).
Natural history	Is a term that describes the normal course of a condition if left untreated.	For instance, we know that 90% of all episodes of acute back pain will have ended within 3–4 weeks – regardless whether we treat them or not. The natural history for many conditions is benign, i.e. they improve no matter what we do – think of the common cold, menstrual pain, injuries, etc.
Negative result	A term commonly used to describe a study where the **experimental treatment** did not generate better outcomes than the control intervention.	Arguably all conclusive results are positive – even knowing that a treatment is not effective is helpful, as patients and clinicians can then choose another one.
Non-experimental study	Is a research project where phenomena are recorded without introducing an experimental treatment.	For instance, recording the outcome of the next 100 back pain patients treated with massage therapy would be a non-experimental study, provided these patients would have received massage therapy anyway.
Non-specific effects	Umbrella term for therapeutic effects which are not caused by the intervention itself but by the circumstances under which they are administered.	Specific and non-specific effects both contribute to the therapeutic response.

Term	Description	Example of use/Comment
Normal distribution	Scatter of data	If data are distributed normally, the **mean** and the **median** are identical.

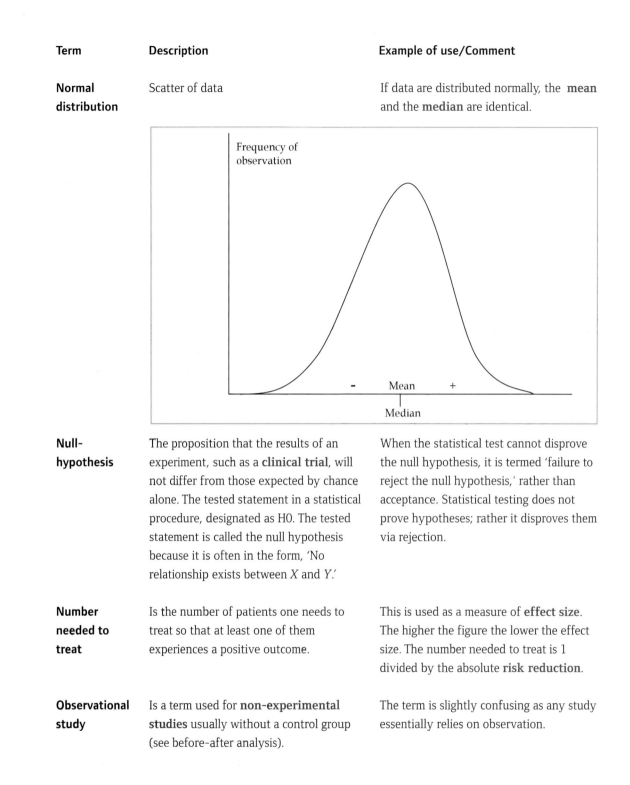

Term	Description	Example of use/Comment
Null-hypothesis	The proposition that the results of an experiment, such as a **clinical trial**, will not differ from those expected by chance alone. The tested statement in a statistical procedure, designated as H0. The tested statement is called the null hypothesis because it is often in the form, 'No relationship exists between X and Y.'	When the statistical test cannot disprove the null hypothesis, it is termed 'failure to reject the null hypothesis,' rather than acceptance. Statistical testing does not prove hypotheses; rather it disproves them via rejection.
Number needed to treat	Is the number of patients one needs to treat so that at least one of them experiences a positive outcome.	This is used as a measure of **effect size**. The higher the figure the lower the effect size. The number needed to treat is 1 divided by the absolute **risk reduction**.
Observational study	Is a term used for **non-experimental studies** usually without a control group (see before-after analysis).	The term is slightly confusing as any study essentially relies on observation.

Term	Description	Example of use/Comment
Odds	Is a measure of the frequency with which an event (such as responding to treatment) occurs in one group compared with how often this event fails to occur.	For instance, if we treat 200 back pain patients with massage therapy and 100 responded and 100 did not respond, the odds for responding could be 100/100 = 1. If, however, with acupuncture 150 responded and 50 did not, the odds would be 150/50 = 3 in favour of acupuncture.
Odds ratio	Is a comparative measure of therapeutic effectiveness.	In the above example, the odds ratio of massage versus acupuncture would equal the ratio of both the above odds: OR = 1/3 = 0.33.
Open-label trial	Is the opposite of a **blind** trial, i.e. a trial where the patient and the therapist know what treatments are being administered.	If, for instance, we conducted a study of massage therapy versus no treatment at all, the patients are obviously aware of receiving treatment and so are the therapists of administering it.
Outcome measure	The term to describe the method by which the results of a study are quantified.	Outcome measures should be: · **appropriate** (e.g. blood pressure for a study in hypertension) · **practicable** (not too difficult to perform) · **reproducible** (give same results on repeat measurements) · **responsive** (sensitive to change in both directions) · **valid** (must quantify what it claims to measure) Outcome measures can relate to different health domains: · **clinical** (e.g. cortisol levels) · **mental** (e.g. ability to concentrate) · **physical** (e.g. range of motion of a joint) · **psychological** (e.g. severity of stress) · **social** (e.g. number of contacts with other individuals) · **spiritual** (e.g. attitude towards life after death)

Term	Description	Example of use/Comment
		When multiple outcomes are recorded, they can be added together to generate an overall index or they can be kept separately to generate a profile.
Parallel group design	This term describes the typical clinical trial where two groups are treated at the same time (in parallel) with two different treatments.	This is contrary to the **cross-over design** where a sequence of treatments is applied, one after the other. It is also different from a study that employs **historical control** where the **experimental group** is compared to patients who have been treated some time before.
Parametric tests	Statistical test which are not based on specific assumptions about the distribution of data.	Parametric tests do not require **normal distribution**.
Peer review	A term used for **critical appraisal** of documents by independent peers.	Grant applications and research articles submitted for publication are usually judged in this way. (See also **reviewer bias**).
Percentile	The proportion of all observations falling between specified values.	For instance, a tertile is the proportion that contains a third of the total data, and there is a lower, middle and an upper tertile. Such data separation can be useful to generate meaningful comparisons. For instance, one could compare the tertile with the highest blood pressure to that with the lowest blood pressure and see whether one is more likely to suffer from a stroke within the next years – this type of research brought to light that high blood pressure is a **risk factor**.

Term	Description	Example of use/Comment
Pharmaco-dynamics	The study of the relationship between dose and effect of a therapy (**dose response**).	One could, for instance, give depressed patients a range of different doses of the herbal antidepressant St John's Wort. This way one might identify the doses that are too low to work, the threshold required for the remedy to work, and the dose where toxic effects occur.
Pharmaco-kinetics	The study of the absorption, distribution and elimination of a drug after administration.	Pharmacokinetic studies are important ways – for instance, they can inform us about the potential of herb-drug interactions.
Phase 1 study	The first investigation of a new treatment in humans. Its particular focus is safety.	These studies are carried out under strictly controlled conditions usually on healthy volunteers.
Phase 2 study	Once phase 1 has been successfully passed, the treatment is tested for **efficacy** under strictly controlled conditions.	Phase 2 studies are usually small and conducted on highly selected patients.
Phase 3 study	The subsequent phase would be to confirm efficacy and test for **effectiveness** in larger patient samples.	In order to get generalisable data, it is essential to test a treatment on large numbers of patients.
Phase 4 study or post marketing (surveillance) study	An exercise to determine how a new treatment performs in everyday clinical practice or see what the long-term effects of it are.	Large numbers and long **follow-ups** are required to see whether rare **adverse-events** are a problem.
Placebo	In clinical trials, placebos or **sham treatments** are often used which are indistinguishable in terms of looks, smell, taste, texture from the **experimental treatment**.	The two main demands on an adequate placebo or sham are that they cannot be distinguished from the experimental treatment and that it has no specific **therapeutic effects**.

Term	Description	Example of use/Comment
Placebo-controlled trial	A trial in which the **experimental group** is compared to a group that receives a placebo intervention.	The aim is to eliminate the influence of placebo-effect on the **outcome** and determine the **specific effects** of the treatment under investigation.
Placebo-effect	Is a non-specific effect caused by the administration of a placebo or sham-treatment.	We often forget that even 'real' treatments generate a placebo-effect in addition to a specific effect.
Population	A group of individuals	If you recruit 50 patients into a clinical trial, they would be your study population.
Positive result	A term commonly used to describe a study where the experimental therapy generated better results than the **control treatment**.	Arguably even studies that do not show the experimental group to be superior are positive if their results are reliable.
Post hoc	Is Latin and means after the event	A post hoc analysis is one which was not originally planned but seemed relevant once a data-set was available. (See also **exploratory analysis**, **data dredging**).
Post-marketing surveillance study	Is an investigation of a treatment which is already in general use (**phase 4 study**). It aims to define how the therapy performs in real life.	The emphasis is often on safety – very large **sample sizes** are required to pick up rare but possibly important adverse effects.
Power	Is a statistical term to describe the reliability by which a study can detect an existing effect.	If a trial has too little power (i.e. the sample size is too small) it can fail to note an effect even though it exists (**false negative** result, **type II error**).
Pragmatic trial	Is a study that, to a large degree, mimics the condition of the real life situation (see also effectiveness trial). Pragmatic trials can incorporate many of the hallmarks of a rigorous study, e.g. they can and usually should be randomised and controlled.	For instance, one could randomise a group of patients into receiving postoperative nursing care in hospital or at home and compare clinical outcomes, cost, patient satisfaction, etc.

Term	Description	Example of use/Comment
Pre-clinical studies	Studies that are not carried out in clinical settings and often not with patients but with human volunteers (**phase I, II study**)	With new drugs, one is understandably keen to prevent harm to patients and test it first under tightly controlled conditions on a small number of volunteers.
Preference trial	Is a study that accounts for patients' preferences and tests the influence of such preferences on the outcome.	For instance, if we conducted a trial of massage versus acupuncture for back pain, some patients might refuse randomization on the grounds that they have a strong preference for one or the other treatment. A preference trial would not **exclude** these patients but **allocate** them to two additional treatment groups. These constitute of patients who elected to have either massage or acupuncture. Such a design would then offer the possibility to compare the outcome (e.g. back pain) of patients who have received the same treatment but were either randomized to it or chose to have it.

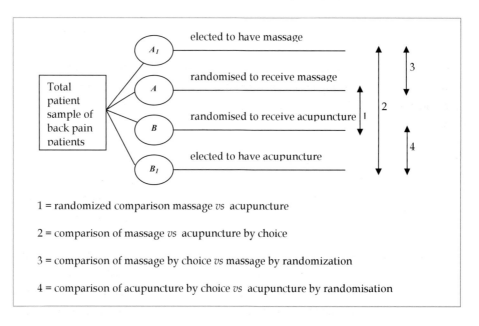

1 = randomized comparison massage *vs* acupuncture

2 = comparison of massage *vs* acupuncture by choice

3 = comparison of massage by choice *vs* massage by randomization

4 = comparison of acupuncture by choice *vs* acupuncture by randomisation

Term	Description	Example of use/Comment
Prevention trial	Most trials test interventions for therapeutic purposes. Studies that focus on preventative measures are called prevention trials.	For instance, one could test the efficacy of Echinacea for treating a common cold or for preventing it. Prevention trials usually require very large sample sizes because the event that is being prevented (e.g. a common cold) occurs only in a fraction of all trial participants. They also need to be long-term, particularly if the event is not immediate – think of prevention of cancer for example. This makes such studies often exceedingly expensive, if not impossible to perform
Primary investigator	The person in charge of the conduct of a research project.	The primary investigator looks after the day to day running of a project and often is the first author on its publication.
Primary outcome measure	This is the endpoint of a study which has been pre-defined in the **protocol** as the outcome of most importance.	Its variability of the primary outcome measure partly determines the **sample size** required for that study. An outcome measure with little variability is body height, for instance – repeated measurements give the same result. An outcome measure with large variability would be the pain intensity upon a stimulus such as manual pressure to a sore muscle.
PRISMA	Is a set of guidelines on how to conduct and publish **systematic reviews** and **meta-analysis** of high quality.	PRIMSA succeeds the QUOROM guidelines which are now obsolete.
Probability	The likelihood of an event occurring (**p-value**).	Statistics cannot give us certainty – they merely provide probabilities with varying degrees of uncertainty.
Prognosis	Is the forecast of a patient's future health.	Prognostic factors such as the age of the patient or the severity of the disease critically influence the results of a study. Therefore it is crucial that, in a controlled clinical trial, the prognosis factors of two

Term	Description	Example of use/Comment
		patients groups are comparable (**randomisation**). Often not all potentially important factors are known. (See also **natural history**).
Prospective study	Is a study where patients are first recruited and studied and subsequently followed into the future (**longitudinal study**).	Imagine a study in which the next 100 depressed patients of one particular practice are treated with massage therapy twice weekly and their symptoms are monitored throughout this period.
Protocol	Is a detailed outline of all necessary details of a research project, such as • the aim • the design • full description of all interventions • inclusion and exclusion criteria • the statistical methods • authorship of any publication	Every research project should have a protocol before it starts – not least because usually an **ethics committee** will want to see and comment on it.
Publication	All research should be published so that others can benefit from it. Researchers have an ethical duty to publish their findings.	There is a saying that 'unpublished research is no research'. If researchers did not publish their results, how could we learn from them? See essay at the end of this book.
Publication bias	See **Bias**.	
P-value	Is a number expressing the **probability** that an observed result occurred by chance.	The conventional p-value which, in medical research, is regarded as statistically significant is 0.05 or 5%. It signifies a 5% probability that a result was due to chance alone.
Qualitative research	Research projects not primarily interested in numerative data. (See also **quantitative research**) but instead in opinions, views, attitudes etc.	Similar to quantitative research, qualitative research should adhere to rigorous standards which can be checked by asking questions such as: • Was the aim of the project clearly specified?

Term	Description	Example of use/Comment
		• Were the methods fully described, adequate and reproductive? • Did the conclusions follow the findings? Qualitative research may help in planning qualitative studies, can be used to generate **hypotheses**, may explain the results of quantitative research. (See also **focus groups**).
Quality adjusted life-years (QALYs)	Combines quality and quantity of life in one index of health benefit.	This allows **comparative cost-utility** analyses across a range of different **outcome measures**.
Quality of life	Describes the state of well-being of an individual.	In different diseases, different factors can affect quality of life. Therefore numerous disease – specific and several generic measures of quality of life have been developed.
Quantitative research	Investigations focused on the generating and assessing numerical data.	The majority of medical research is quantitative. Researchers usually insist on reliable figures about phenomena, outcomes, etc.
Random	Means 'by chance'.	Random allocation or randomization is used in clinical trials to make sure that all characteristics of two groups except the one under investigation are similar. Random error is error which occurs by chance. Researchers also speak of 'background noise'.
Randomised clinical trial (RCT)	Is a **clinical trial** where patients are allocated by chance to one of several (usually two) treatment groups.	The simplest way of randomizing is flipping a coin, but computer programs can achieve randomisation more elegantly. Subsequently patients are treated and eventually the outcomes of both groups are compared. Frequently the term 'randomised controlled trial' is used synonymously; as there cannot be a

Term	Description	Example of use/Comment

randomised trial without a control group, this term may be less meaningful.

The RCT is generally regarded as the design that minimises **bias** most effectively.

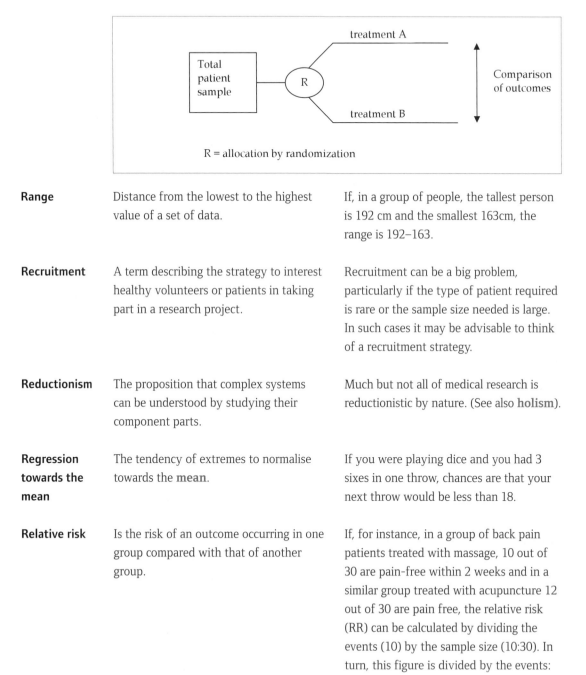

R = allocation by randomization

Term	Description	Example of use/Comment
Range	Distance from the lowest to the highest value of a set of data.	If, in a group of people, the tallest person is 192 cm and the smallest 163cm, the range is 192–163.
Recruitment	A term describing the strategy to interest healthy volunteers or patients in taking part in a research project.	Recruitment can be a big problem, particularly if the type of patient required is rare or the sample size needed is large. In such cases it may be advisable to think of a recruitment strategy.
Reductionism	The proposition that complex systems can be understood by studying their component parts.	Much but not all of medical research is reductionistic by nature. (See also **holism**).
Regression towards the mean	The tendency of extremes to normalise towards the **mean**.	If you were playing dice and you had 3 sixes in one throw, chances are that your next throw would be less than 18.
Relative risk	Is the risk of an outcome occurring in one group compared with that of another group.	If, for instance, in a group of back pain patients treated with massage, 10 out of 30 are pain-free within 2 weeks and in a similar group treated with acupuncture 12 out of 30 are pain free, the relative risk (RR) can be calculated by dividing the events (10) by the sample size (10:30). In turn, this figure is divided by the events:

Term	Description	Example of use/Comment
		sample size (12:30) for the comparator for treatment. RR = 10:30 ÷ 12:30 = 0.83 If the outcomes in both groups were the same, the RR would be 1. The more it deviates from 1, the greater the difference in outcome between the groups.
Reliability	Is the extent to which repeated measurements agree with each other.	Diagnostic tests need to be reliable to be useful.
Research question	Every good research project must have a clear research question or **hypothesis**. The question should be important and answerable with the proposed methodology. In other words, the research question and the study design need to be well-matched.	We want to determine the efficacy of a treatment the **clinical trial** is a good method. If we want to know how many people use CAM, a good **survey** might be adequate. If we want to find out why they use CAM, an **interview study** or **focus group** could be the right methodology. An example of a good research question could be, for instance, does the use of a water bed prevent pressure sores in permanently bed-ridden patients.
Retrospective study	Is a study that is designed to look back in time; the events of interest for such a study have already taken place. The opposite is a **prospective study**.	For instance, we might decide to assess the outcome of all patients of the last two years treated with acupuncture compared with those treated without acupuncture by studying case note.
Risk-benefit concept	The notion that, in absolute terms, neither the benefit nor the risk of a therapy are crucial, but only information on both can lead to wise (therapeutic) decisions.	Put simply: a recommendable treatment must do more good than harm. If a treatment generates only small benefits, even minor risks count heavily.

Term	Description	Example of use/Comment
Risk-benefit ratio (or balance or profile)	This describes an attempt to set the risks of a therapy in relation to its benefits.	Even though the word 'ratio' implies a neat calculation, things are usually too complex for that. Information may be incomplete and the risk may be difficult to compare to the benefit. For instance, if 500 of 1000 back pain patients are helped by spinal manipulation (i.e. the benefit) and 1 of 1000 suffers a severe adverse effect as a consequence of that treatment (i.e. the risk), how do we put the risks in relation to the benefit? Usually this is a clinical judgement rather that an exact science. If, by such a judgement, the risks of a therapy seem to outweigh its benefit, it cannot be recommended for clinical routine. If, for instance, a therapy generates only marginal benefit, even relatively minor risks might tilt the risk-benefit balance into the negative area. On the other hand, most of us would accept considerable risks of a treatment such as chemotherapy for cancer, where the benefit is potentially huge, i.e. a life may be saved.
Risk-factor	Is a factor that negatively affects the **probability** of an event to occur.	Well-studied risk factors include hypertension which increases the likelihood of a stroke, hypercholesterol-aemia which increases the likelihood of a heart attack, and smoking which increases the likelihood of cancer and cardiovascular diseases. Hypertension and hypercholesterolaemia can be treated, they are therefore changeable risk factors. Other risk factors cannot be altered e.g. the family history or the age of a patient.

Term	Description	Example of use/Comment
Sample size	Is the number of patients included in a study.	If the sample size of a clinical trial is too small, a real effect may be overlooked (**type II error, false negative**). If it is too large, patients' cooperation and good will as well as money may have been spent unnecessarily (**mega-trials**). The optimal sample size of a clinical trial depends on a range of factors such as level of **significance** one aims for and the variability of the **outcome measure**.
Sampling error	Occurs if a particular group of study participants is not representative of the whole population from which it is drawn.	For instance, we might study the level of stress in nurses in our hospital and find that 20% suffer from it. But this finding might not be representative for all nurses in the country. The stress level could be higher or lower in other settings.
Selection	Allocation of patients in a clinical trial to a treatment group through a process of choice; the choosing can be done by the clinician or by the patient.	Selection of this type inevitably leads to selection bias which, in turn, leads to unreliable results. This can be overcome by allocation through randomisation.
Selection bias	See **Bias**.	
Selective reporting	Regrettably a common phenomenon in research; authors sometimes only report data they like and 'forget' about those they don't like.	This can generate a false overall impression and biased conclusions of **systematic reviews**.
Sensitivity	Each diagnostic test should be accurate. In order to be accurate it has to be both sensitive and specific. Sensitivity is a measure of the proportion of patients with condition x testing positive with a test that aims to diagnose that condition.	Is kinesiology an accurate test for food allergy? If we test 400 individuals who suffer from food allergy, we might generate the following results: test positive: 100 test negative: 300 The sensitivity (S) of this test can be calculated $S = 100 \div (300 + 100) = 0.25$ This means the test will only correctly identify 25% of the patients suffering from food allergy.

Term	Description	Example of use/Comment
Sham	For non-drug treatments there usually is no placebo intervention for conducting **placebo-controlled trials**. But, in some cases, one can design a sham intervention that serves the same purpose as a placebo.	For instance, for acupuncture studies, researchers have created a range of sham-acupuncture treatments, e.g. sticking the needle in non-acupuncture points.
Side-effect	Is any effect of a treatment that is unexpected.	The term is often used synonymous with **adverse effect**. Strictly speaking, however, side-effects can also be positive. For instance, a nurse receiving relaxation training for stress-reduction may find that her stress level is reduced but also her sleep has improved and her concentration is better. The latter two effects might be seen as side-effects.
Sign	Objective characteristic of an illness or clinical state of a patient, objective evidence of a disease. (See also **symptom**).	A sign for diabetes, for instance, is an elevated blood sugar level after fasting.
Significance	Statistical significance is the probability of rejecting the **null hypothesis** when, in reality, it is true.	Clinical significance is a judgment call deciding what effect we regard as **clinically relevant**.
Single-blind trial	Is a trial where only one party is unaware of the group allocation.	For instance, acupuncture trials can be single-blind if the patient cannot distinguish a sham (placebo) intervention from real acupuncture. The therapist will, however, be aware of that difference. Such a study would be categorised as single-blind. (See also **double blind**).
Social desirability	If we are kind to patients, they tend to be kind to us. This may mean that many claim to suffer less severe symptoms, even if there was no improvement at all. This phenomenon or **artefact** can affect the results of clinical trials exaggerating the effect of a therapy, particularly if the **outcome measure** is a subjective one such as pain or depression.	Probably the best way to eliminate this factor in clinical trials is to have a control group in which social desirability plays the same role as in the **experimental group**. In this case, the **inter-group difference** would be unaffected. This is achieved with patient-blinded, controlled clinical trials. The inter-group comparison of the results should then be devoid of any confounding by social desirability.

Term	Description	Example of use/Comment
Specific effects	Specific effects are those directly caused by the therapy rather than by circumstances in which it is given.	The total therapeutic response of a therapy is typically due to **specific** and **non-specific** effects.
Specificity	Any diagnostic test must have an **acceptable sensitivity** and specificity, in order to be accurate. Specificity is a measure of the proportion of patients free of the condition in question, who are correctly identified with a diagnostic test as not having that condition.	For instance, if we test 600 patients suffering from a food allergy with kinesiology, we might generate the following results. test positive: 400 test negative: 200 The specificity (Sp) of this test can be calculated $Sp = 200 \div (200 + 400) = 0.34$ In other words, the test will correctly identify 34% of healthy patients as being without the condition.
Sponsor	This term is often used in two different ways. Firstly, it can describe the organisation which finances a research project. Secondly, it can denote the institution that is ultimately responsible for it.	If I conducted a clinical trial of St John's wort supported by a herbal manufacturer, that firm would be my financial sponsor while my university would be the academic sponsor.
Standard deviation	The absolute value of the average difference of individual values from the **mean**.	The term describes the variability of data within a set of data and is often used when statistical data are presented.
Statistical power	Is the likelihood of detecting a statistically significant difference, if a difference does actually exist, or that the **null-hypothesis** is rejected if, in fact, it is false.	The statistical power depends on a range of factors. • the **sample size** • the nature of the **outcome measure**) • the **confidence interval** used.
Superiority trials	**Clinical trials** can test whether two treatments generate similar results (**equivalence trial**) or whether one is superior to another, e.g. **placebo**.	The latter is much more common.

Term	Description	Example of use/Comment
Surrogate endpoint	Endpoints that are relatively easy to measure and stand for endpoints which are not measurable.	It has been wryly noted that, in medicine, we tend to measure what is measurable rather that what is desirable. Often the things we really want to know are not readily quantifiable. For instance, if we eat less animal fat, do we suffer fewer heart attacks? To study this question in a clinical trial would be difficult, not least because we would require a study with a **follow-up** of several decades. But as we know that certain characteristics, such as elevated levels of cholesterol, are **risk factors** for heart attacks, we might investigate whether eating less animal fat lowers cholesterol levels. This would then be a surrogate endpoint. In other words, a surrogate endpoint or **outcome measure** is a marker that relates to the ultimately most important outcome which is not readily measurable.
Symptom	Characteristic of an illness as expressed by the patients own sensations and feelings. (See also **sign**).	A symptom of upper respiratory tract infection, for instance, is a runny nose.
Syndrome	The totality of **symptoms**.	Metabolic syndrome, for instance, is characterised by overweight, impaired insulin tolerance and elevated blood levels of certain tests.
Synergism	The combined effect of two or more processes which exceed the effect of their individual actions.	Herbal medicines are claimed to act synergistically through several pharmacologically active compounds.
Systematic review	This is a transparent and reproducible summary of the totality of the evidence available on a certain subject. Systematic reviews provide more accurate information than single studies.	For instance, if we needed to know whether massage therapy is effective in relieving acute back pain, it might be tempting to simply review the few studies we are aware of. That might create a false impression. To minimise bias, we should consider not part of but all the available evidence.

Term	Description	Example of use/Comment
Therapeutic encounter	Interactions between a therapist and a patient.	It can have effects of its own which are classified as **non-specific effects** or context effects. In clinical trials, these effects can influence the results and mimic the specific effects of a treatment.
Therapy	Treatment of illnesses	Therapy can be pharmacological, physical, or psychological.
Toxicity	The poisonous properties of substances and drugs.	Most chemicals have toxicity when taken in large **doses** – even natural ones.
Type I error	Is the mistake we make if we do not accept a result which, in fact, is true.	For instance, if we conducted a clinical trial comparing two pure placebos, there should be no difference in outcome. But our study could be biased and produce a **false positive result**. This would be a type I error.
Type II error	Is the mistake we make if we accept a result which, in fact, is not true.	For instance, we might conduct a trial of acupuncture for knee osteoarthritis versus sham acupuncture and find no difference in outcome. But our study might have been too small to be able to generate a significant difference between the two groups. Thus a true effect has been overlooked and we have produced a **false negative result**. This would be a type II error.
Validity	Outcome measures and questionnaires should be valid i.e. achieve what we hope they do.	There are several ways of checking validity • face validity essentially means using one's common sense, i.e. does this seem ok on the face of it? • content validity checks whether all important areas are covered; this can be achieved by exploratory interviews, discussions, focus groups etc.

Term	Description	Example of use/Comment
		• construct validity checks whether the questionnaire or outcome measure corresponds to what people understand by a certain construct. For instance, if the question is about quality of life, it is important that researchers and patients attach the same meaning to the term • criterion validity means comparing one measure or questionnaire against an existing 'gold standard'
Variance	The variability around the mean within a set of data	All data sets have a degree of variability which can occur naturally and can be caused by **non-accurate** measurement for instance.
Verum	Is a Latin term for real; in research it is often used to describe the **experimental treatment**.	For instance, in a trial of acupuncture versus sham-acupuncture, the former would be the verum.
Visual analogue scale	This is a simple measure for subjective symptoms such as pain.	Essentially the patient is asked to indicate on a line between no pain and maximum pain their current or past pain level. Subsequently this can be used for quantifying pain or other symptoms.

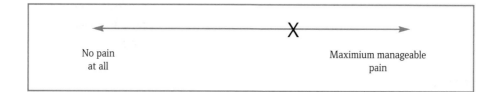

Term	Description	Example of use/Comment
Washout period	In **crossover trials** patients are treated first with one treatment and subsequently with another. This means the effects of the first should have subsided before the other can start. The interim period required to achieve this is called washout period (**carry-over effects**).	The graph depicts this schematically.

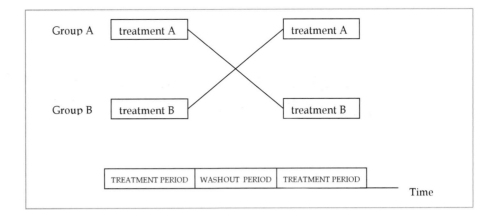

Term	Description	Example of use/Comment
Withdrawal	In a **clinical trial**, some patients may need to be removed, for example, because, they develop **adverse effects** or do not **comply** with the protocol.	Different from **dropouts** who are patients failing to show up.
Yellow card scheme	A scheme by national drug regulatory agencies to report adverse effects of treatments. These are then recorded and can provide valuable information about the safety of these interventions.	The UK yellow card scheme has proved to be a powerful tool to identifying safety problems for licensed drugs. In CAM there usually is no such monitoring system which is why our knowledge about safety may be incomplete.

CHAPTER 6 FREQUENTLY ASKED QUESTIONS AND COMMON MISCONCEPTIONS

This short chapter lists many of the questions I have been asked about research, especially in non-medical contexts. The responses given are those I have come to believe are true.

1. **Many therapies do not aim at a cure of a disease but at aiding a recovery, reducing pain, stress etc or at maintaining motivation while other treatments are administered. How can these effects be shown in a clinical trial?**
   This is simply a question of **outcome measure**. If you are interested in a cure then you measure cure rates. If you are interested in motivation, pain, stress etc, you need to quantify these qualities.

2. **How many patients does one need for a clinical trial?**
   There is no such thing as an adequate **sample size** for all studies. The optimal sample size depends on several factors including **variability** of the **outcome measure**, the **significance level** and the **power** of a study. If the sample size is too small, one is in danger of missing an effect which does exist, i.e. committing a **type II error**.

3. **Placebo-controlled trials are often not a realistic option because there is no placebo, think of massage, for instance – what is the solution?**
   True, for many treatments, there is no adequate **placebo**. In such cases, the **experimental treatment** could be tested against a 'gold standard' or against no treatment at all.

4. **Patients may not want to be randomised to one of two treatment groups – is there a solution to this problem?**

Yes, one can, for instance, design a controlled clinical trial with **preference groups** (preference trial). In such a study, patients who do not mind being randomised are randomised, those who have a preference for either treatment A or B may select these options.

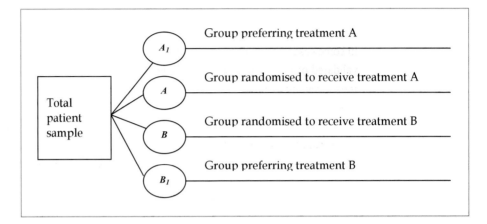

5. **In CAM, treatments are often highly individualised – does that defy testing them in clinical trials?**

No, it is always possible to allocate patients (by randomisation or other means) to two groups. One would receive the individualised treatment and the control group would receive another therapy, for instance, placebo or treatment as usual. Such studies exist, for instance, in homeopathy or traditional herbalism where individualisation is often considered essential.

6. **Surely, if a patient experiences a benefit from a certain intervention, we do not need a trial to inform us that it is effective**

If a patient or a clinician observes a benefit, this could be due to a specific effect of the therapy but it could also be caused by a range of other factors called context or non-specific effects, e.g:

·   **Hawthorne effect**
·   **natural history of the condition**
·   **placebo-effect**
·   **regression towards the mean**
·   **social desirability**

For optimal outcome, patients should benefit from both specific and non specific effects.

7. **Many forms of CAM have been around for hundreds of years – does that not guarantee efficacy and safety?**

   Sadly not, it renders efficacy and safety perhaps more likely but it is certainly no guarantee. There are many examples of treatments which were perceived as effective or safe for many years and only proper testing revealed that this was an illusion. An ancient example is blood letting and a recent one is hormone replacement therapy.

8. **In research, one always measures parameters like blood pressure or cholesterol; surely these outcomes do not capture the holistic nature of CAM?**

   In some cases, this may be true. But, on the other hand, there are certainly many validated **outcome measures** which do capture this – think of **quality of life measures**, for instance.

9. **Research results are not very relevant to real life practice. Have they ever influenced the way we treat real patients?**

   Ever since healthcare has become scientific – around 150 years ago – our treatments have become immeasurably better and our diagnoses hugely more reliable. Consequently the health of the population has improved remarkably. Real life practice has changed fundamentally and real patients benefit significantly from this progress.

10. **The principles of evidence-based medicine may seem quite logical – except that clinicians don't have 'evidence-based patients', they have real human beings with very complex problems.**

    It is true that patients are invariably complex individuals with complex problems that often don't fit in our neat scientific categories. Science is only slowly coping with this level of complexity. But much of the evidence that already exists can be used to the benefit of even complex cases. And complex cases can be handled better if we consider the existing medical knowledge. The alternative would be to not apply evidence at all and this would certainly be counterproductive. In my experience, the argument ('my patients are not evidence-based') is often used by clinicians who are not capable of applying existing knowledge correctly. Sadly, the ones who suffer are the patients.

11. **Patients who opt for CAM are generally not in favour of science; they may not want to participate in clinical trials. Is CAM-research feasible under these circumstances?**

    In certain settings, some patients may refuse to volunteer for a trial. But research does not have to take place in such settings. There are some situations which are well suited for clinical service and others are well suited for clinical research. If one particular setting is not ideal for answering a certain question, it should be perhaps answered in another one.

12. **Research is very expensive but CAM is a relatively poor field. Therefore we cannot do research in this area.**

Yes, research is expensive and CAM does not have the equivalent of a rich pharmaceutical industry that sponsors much of medical research. It is therefore crucial that the few funding sources that do exist in CAM are used optimally; these include, for instance, the research councils, patient organisations, practitioner organisations, charities, private benefactors. At present, these sources are not always used to their full potential.

13. **'Big Pharma' is out to suppress CAM; whatever we do, we will be ignored or worse.**

I have no reason to believe this is true – but I would be interested to receive evidence showing that I am wrong.

14. **Aren't the big healthcare decisions taken on a political level where evidence counts very little?**

If we look how healthcare has changed during the last 50 years or so, I think no one can deny that scientific evidence has played a major role in changing it to the better. I admit that, on a political level, other considerations are important too, but sound evidence will eventually always win the day.

15. **Clinical trials tell us nothing about an individual patient. But clinicians treat individuals. Are trials really that important?**

If you only want to know about one single patient you can always conduct an '**individual patient trial**'. But usually we are interested in findings which are reproducible and can be **generalised**. If things are not reproducible they tell us nothing about the next patient who comes through our door. Even clinicians who emphasize the uniqueness of each patient generalise from one patient to another. Clinical trials tell us about the likelihood with which a patient may benefit from a given therapy. It is impossible to deny, I think, that this constitutes valuable information.

16. **Why do clinical trials often take so long?**

It is true that, from the initial planning period to the final publication of the results, clinical trials can take many months. This has many reasons. For instance, it can take a long time to recruit sufficiently large numbers. Some trials require a follow-up of several years, even after treatment has stopped.

17. **Our medical wards are full of people suffering from adverse effects of conventional drugs. I have never seen a single patient with adverse effects of CAM. Why then is it important to research the safety of CAM?**

We should think of therapeutic benefits and risks in terms of balance. If the benefits of a treatment are unknown or minor, even small risks can tilt the balance. This may well be the case for much of CAM. To make sure that we are not exposing patients to treatments with negative risk-benefit balance, we need to research safety issues thoroughly.

18. **Let's be honest: many conventional treatments are also not evidence-based, so why insist that we conduct research to make CAM evidence-based?**

There are two answers to that question. Firstly, the best evidence I know of suggests that 90% of what happens in primary care is based on sound evidence. If we don't want double standards, then we should work towards a similar figure also in CAM. Secondly, even if conventional medicine were not evidence-based at all, CAM should be – if many people are killed on our roads each year, this is no reason to be in favour of unsafe trains!

19. **An old saying holds that today's fallacies are tomorrow's wisdom. So perhaps CAM is the healthcare of the future?**

True some innovations were ridiculed when they first emerged. The telephone, for instance, was initially thought to be a most useless gadget. But surely that does not mean that everything we today look upon as silly will be useful tomorrow. Innovations have to be proven to be useful, and, in medicine, this is best done with research.

20. **CAM gives something to patients that conventional medicine does not provide. This is obvious, and we need no research to know that.**

If that is so obvious, then research would confirm it. But perhaps patients are just bamboozled into thinking CAM is helpful. In any case, if that 'something' is real, we should define what it is and let all patients benefit from it. The way to achieve this is through proper research.

21. **If we research CAM, we would only be playing the game by biomedicine's rules. In the end, this would destroy CAM.**

No, 'biomedicine's rules' are not rules, they are simply common sense applied to healthcare. What counts is not obeying some imaginary laws but defining what is most helpful for patients. The best way to do this is to conduct research that answers important questions.

22. **Research is by definition reductionist – but CAM is holistic. So CAM research is nonsense.**

Most research is reductionist. But that does not mean that one cannot adapt the methods such that the holistic nature of CAM is accounted for. In my experience, this is usually feasible with a bit of expertise and will.

23. **There is evidence that clinicians will follow their 'informed intuition' and experience even if they are not in line with the results of scientific research. So why conduct research in the first place?**

There may be good reasons why, in a certain instance, clinicians do things that are not evidence-based. But these instances surely are the exception and not the rule.

24. **Clinical trials create a very artificial situation which has often nothing to do with real life. Can clinical trials really tell us anything useful for everyday practice?**

One can design a study such that it reflects 'real life' very well. Such studies are called **pragmatic trials**, and they can tell us useful things about clinical practice.

25. **Sometimes one gets the impression that some researchers have the agenda to discredit CAM – so why should we cooperate with them?**

If that were true, you are right: don't cooperate. But I think, in the vast majority of cases that impression is not correct.

26. **CAM research is merely an attempt to appropriate and transform our treatments. We should be very cautious because the CAM practitioner will be left behind with nothing!**

This is not what good research is about. It is about finding the best ways to help as many patients as possible. Research is not a 'turf war' and good researchers are not seeking to win any battles.

27. **Some treatments include a sheer endless range of different modalities. Take aromatherapy, for instance. Surely we cannot submit every oil in every dilution to clinical trials?**

Perhaps not. But we can do a **randomised clinical trial** where say 50 patients with one condition (e.g. premenstrual stress) are treated by one of say 10 therapists who are very experienced and do what their experience tells them. The control group could at the same time have conventional care. At the end of the treatment period, we compare the results (e.g. stress level) of both groups.

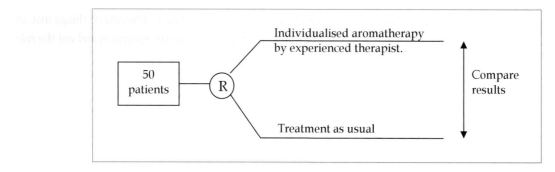

This study would not be a test of this or that oil but of aromatherapy as a whole.

CHAPTER 7   **FINAL THOUGHTS**

This concluding section of the book has the aim of re-emphasising a range of important issues: causality, bias, placebo, and evidence-based medicine. It ends with some advice that might come in handy for all those readers who may be considering publishing an article in a medical journal. Some of the issues are of fundamental importance for understanding research – and they are often misunderstood by CAM practitioners. The following essays will, I hope, be helpful in setting the record straight.

Causality, merely an obsession of scientists?

Clinicians are sometimes puzzled by scientists' insistence on asking questions about cause and effect. They claim that reductionistic concepts of this type are not applicable to clinical medicine, particularly not to CAM where things are so subtle and complex that the 'naivety' of precise linear thinking is counter-productive. They may claim that CAM, nursing and some 'talking' therapies are 'holistic' and so not suited to precise causality. I beg to differ and will use the example of a recent research paper to explain why.

Norwegian Study

Norwegian researchers recorded the CAM usage of cancer patients. Essentially they confirmed what others had shown before: some patients do and some don't use CAM. Subsequently this population was followed up and the fate of all patients was recorded.

This generated a truly surprising result. Those participants who used CAM lived on average for a shorter time than those who did not. In principle, such a finding is compatible with at least two dramatically different interpretations:

i)   CAM-use caused early death.

ii)   Other factors associated with CAM-use caused early death.

To say that causation is irrelevant would be like claiming it does not matter which of the two interpretations is correct; surely anyone trying CAM will want to know whether this will cause them to die prematurely! So surely clinicians need to know that too. In other words: causality does matter.

Establishing causality

So how can we establish causality? How can we find out which of the two interpretations is correct? Six criteria have long been well-established for assessing the likelihood of cause effect relationships:

i)   the observed phenomenon should be **biologically plausible**

ii)   the **association** should be specific

iii)   it should be consistent

iv)   the time frame must be logical

v)   the association should have sufficient strength

vi)   there should be a **dose-responsive relationship**.

If this sounds technical or complicated, don't worry; it isn't, and I will take you through it step by step.

Plausibility

In the case of the Norwegian study, one might argue that some forms of CAM are burdened with risks that could hasten death; such risks have repeatedly been described. For instance, there is a reasonable suspicion that some herbal medicines or other natural supplements might impede the action of chemotherapy. If this is true, taking such remedies would hasten death.

Alternatively one might assume that, in some cases, using CAM treatments means giving up life-saving conventional therapies. This, in turn, could be responsible for premature deaths. Thus the biological plausibility of CAM being a causal factor in the Norwegian study clearly could exist – at least theoretically.

Association

Specificity of association, in the above example, means that only CAM use, and not some other associated factor, is linked with early deaths. Researchers must therefore always scrutinise their data very carefully to exclude the influence of any other variables of potential importance. We can only be sure about specificity, if that is done thoroughly. The obvious problem is that most data sets are limited, and one can never make conclusions about factors that have not been assessed in the first place.

In the case of the Norwegian study, an associated factor could be severity of disease. Perhaps the more ill patients are, the higher is the likelihood that they try CAM?

Consistency

Consistency of the observation is equally important; it is one of the reasons why scientists insist on **independent replications** of any new findings. If an observed phenomenon (e.g. CAM-users die earlier) is based on a causal relationship it will show up over and over again. If researchers in the UK or elsewhere repeated the Norwegian study, would they obtain a similar result?

In the absence of **consistency** of an association, the observed phenomenon might well be an **artefact** of some unknown **confounding factor**. Or, in extreme cases, it could be due to someone cheating – after all, researchers – even scientists are only human!

Time frame

It is obvious that the cause has to precede the event; temporal correctness of the association is thus an essential and logical precondition for causality.

This was the lesson an intriguing Italian study recently brought home quite clearly. In this experiment, some patients' charts were submitted to 'energy healing' years after these patients had been dismissed from hospital.

The researchers then analysed the time each patient had stayed in hospital. Patients whose charts received the healing turned out to be associated with shorter hospital stays than those whose charts were left untouched. This study is an excellent example of the importance of temporal correctness; this factor alone can sometimes demonstrate the absurdity of a result.

The Italian study was an amusing hoax to teach us a lesson. In the case of the Norwegian study, however, CAM treatments occurred obviously before death. Thus, based on this criterion, causality would be a possibility.

Strength of association

The strength of an association describes the size and the robustness of the effect. In the Norwegian study, 79% of the CAM users and 65% of the non-users died during the 8-year follow-up period. The effect was **statistically significant** but it is difficult to estimate the strength of the association using this data alone.

Dose response (frequency of treatment)

Dose-response relationships are excellent indicators of causality. Did patients who used CAM once a month live longer than those who used CAM once a week, and did that group live on average longer than those patients who used CAM on a daily basis?

Similarly, one could ask whether patients who used 10 types of CAM died earlier than those who employed 5 forms of CAM, and longer than those who only used one type of CAM. If an increase of one factor increases the effect, that factor becomes a likely candidate for being the cause of the effect.

Causality matters

All of this shows, I think, that causality matters – not just for academics in their 'ivory towers' but also in a real and practical way. Causality must be assessed systematically and such an assessment usually is essential for understanding what is going on. In many instances, this evaluation will open new relevant questions that may need further research.

With the Norwegian study, for instance, one would want to conduct a careful analysis according to disease severity. As I mentioned above, it is possible (even likely) that CAM-users were more severely diseased than non-users (they could, for instance, have tried CAM because of desperation with the severity of their cancer).

If that were true, the association between CAM-use and early death would have failed the specificity test – thus it would probably not reflect a cause-effect relationship. Consider all of this, and then try to argue against the importance of assessing causality – I don't think you can.

Bias, the stuff of a researcher's nightmare

Bias is a prepossession with something so that the mind does not respond impartially to it. Bias, in other words, clouds our judgement.

Therefore, in research, we need to get rid of it where we can and the best we can. Bias is to the researcher, what weeds are for the gardener. Bias seems to be everywhere and it certainly dies hard.

There are now several conditions for which acupuncture and/or herbal medicines have been proven to work according to the rules of evidence-based medicine. Why then are they not being adopted in mainstream healthcare? The answer can be summarised in one word: bias.

Thus all of us who work in CAM are acutely aware and endlessly frustrated by the ill effects of bias. Bias is not just a hindrance to objectivity of scientific debates, it can harm people! Bias even kills. If that is the case, why are we often blind to our own biases?

Types of bias

Publication bias, for instance, cuts both ways. Major CAM journals publish virtually nothing but positive results. Either there are only positive findings to report or something is seriously amiss – the latter seems much more likely.

Again, such bias is real and can lead to tangible harm. Several research studies have shown that the advice provided by consumer books on CAM is often not reliable and sometimes outright irresponsible. In extreme cases, it can be a risk factor to the health of the reader. The potential for harm is obvious.

Bias is everywhere, and takes many guises. A recently published list included 45 different types of bias. 'Investigator bias' was not amongst them. But I suggest that, in medical research, investigator bias is hugely important.

Our working definition for it is that bias in research is due to a **conflict of interest** resulting from passionate beliefs held by the investigators. Strictly speaking, such a conflict requires declaration. The reality is, however, that it is never laid open. Investigator bias can influence all stages of a research project.

From the very outset it can influence the general attitude towards the project. Research is at its best when it tests **hypotheses**. The biased researcher, however, has strong beliefs and is likely to approach a project in order to 'prove' a point.

Testing and 'proving'

The difference between testing and proving is considerable. A researcher who is convinced of the value of a particular treatment might misuse science as an alibi to demonstrate the efficacy of his therapy. Similarly, an investigator with a preconceived negative attitude toward a particular intervention might set out to disprove its efficacy.

A major source of investigator bias may thus be introduced even before a trial is designed. What research question does the investigator ask? The precise **hypothesis** tested for a particular intervention clearly affects the likelihood of a positive outcome.

An intervention may be more likely to succeed if tested in patients suffering a particular ailment at a particular stage of the disease course.

- 'Does relaxation therapy prolong survival in terminally-ill cancer patients', or
- 'Does relaxation therapy improve the quality of their remaining life?

Different **research questions** can generate dramatically different answers about the value of one and the same therapy.

The planning period of a **clinical trial** provides further room for bias. It is not difficult to conceive a study of an ineffective treatment that is more than likely to generate a **false positive result**, i.e. suggesting the effectiveness of the ineffective intervention.

One could, for instance, compare it to a therapy that causes the **outcome measures** to worsen.

The **inter-group comparison** would subsequently yield an apparent advantage in the **experimental group**.

In the opposite direction, a trial could compare the effect of a herbal with a conventional anti-depressant to treat patients with intractable depression, showing that both fail equally and conclude that the herbal medicine does not work. This is not far fetched at all; in fact such a study was published not long ago in a leading medical journal.

Investigators have considerable scope to influence the likelihood that a trial will give a positive or negative result through their choice of **outcome measure** and design of key features of the research protocol.

Large changes may be more likely with 'soft' measures such as questionnaire-based variables than with 'hard' outcomes such as blood tests or body weight. If the former are combined with an inadequate **control procedure**, or with inadequate **blinding** of subjects and assessors, then false-positive result is pre-programmed.

We know that engendering expectations of benefit from a particular intervention can produce dramatic effects in patients through a **placebo response**. Even if subjects are adequately blinded as to whether they receive **verum** or placebo treatment, the expectations of the non-blinded experimenter can be conveyed to the patient. Bias may also be introduced at the measurement stage if the assessor is not blinded to **patient allocation**.

Bias in evaluation and writing up

Perhaps the largest scope for bias exists during the phase when the results are being evaluated. One obvious way of producing a false positive result is **data dredging** or fishing for a significant result: if the primary **outcome measure** of a trial does not show what one had hoped, one simply carries on looking until, Bingo, one parameter yields **statistical significance**. The published article might then imply that the highlighted result relates to the most important outcome measure.

Once the results are on the table, they need writing up. This phase of the research project offers numerous further opportunities for introducing bias.

Negative results may be interpreted as being (almost) positive. The abstract, the section that most people read, could be 'economical with the truth'.

Choosing which results to report strongly affects the 'spin' on the final research report. A common failing, particularly in abstracts, is to report only the positive findings among a larger number of outcome measures. The consequence of such a scenario would be a false overall impression. In other words, biased reporting misleads the reader.

There are numerous subtle ways for the biased investigator to mislead us. The above examples only describe the tip of the iceberg. For the unsuspecting reader of a research paper, all of this can be undetectable. The published article might reveal little or nothing of the bias that distorted it. Often one needs insider knowledge or considerable detective skills to uncover bias.

The obvious way to minimise investigator bias is to ensure that only properly trained people do the research. The best protection against it is a good dose of scepticism and critical evaluation. And this is precisely what much of this book is about.

Placebo-effect: a complex and often misunderstood phenomenon

Before powerful and effective drugs were beginning to emerge some hundred years ago, clinicians relied almost entirely on the amazing effects of placebos. They tended to falsely attribute any therapeutic success thus achieved to the 'specific' actions of their prescriptions. But placebo effects are part of the response to (almost) any treatment (even the most effective ones). Researchers are usually fascinated with specific effects and often they are disinterested in the complex issues surrounding the placebo-effect.

Defining placebo

So what is a placebo? It used to be described simply as 'make believe medicine' or 'medicine of convenience'; the word placebo means 'to please'. Today there are numerous elaborate definitions but, to keep things simple, it can be described as the form of a therapy without its content.

Most physicians have amusing stories about placebo effects. Mine dates back to the days when I was still at medical school. I had been taught to wire up patients for electrocardiograms. One of my very first patients, an elderly lady with ischaemic heart disease, gave me a tip after I had done her test (the first money I ever earned in medicine!) and said with a smile 'Thank you that was great, I feel so much better, my chest pain has completely gone'. This story still makes me smile, but it tells us more about placebo than is apparent at first glance.

It would be fascinating to define why placebo effects are sometimes powerful and on other occasions almost totally absent. This seems to depend on the type of treatment. An invasive or in other ways impressive procedure is likely to induce stronger effects than a simple pill. My patient was obviously impressed with the 'high tech' atmosphere of being wired up to a sophisticated piece of testing equipment, not realising that it had no curative effect.

There are studies showing that sham surgery (opening the skin without doing the actual operation) can bring pain relief to nearly 100% of the patients. Surgeons won't like this, but surgery invariably comes with a powerful placebo response.

Acupuncture is another example: it is invasive in that it entails puncturing the skin, and some trials show that close to 100% of pain sufferers benefit from a sham-acupuncture.

Patient expectation

Furthermore, the response will depend on the patient. The higher the expectation, the stronger the effect. Obviously, the elderly lady in my story was full of expectation. Involving the patient in the therapy will also enhance the placebo-effect. In a controlled clinical trial with patients suffering from varicose veins, we have shown that a placebo-pill is less beneficial than a placebo-cream. The cream has to be rubbed on to the skin and the patient therefore gets actively involved in the treatment which, in turn, seems to yield a better outcome.

Therapist expectation

The expectation of the therapist seems similarly crucial. It will determine the interaction with the patient which conceivably influences the therapeutic success. When I did the electrocardiogram, I certainly tried to make up with kindness and understanding what I lacked in experience. Doctors who believe in a given remedy have more success with it than those who are more sceptical about it. Similarly, a positive encounter with the patient can increase the success rate by as much as 100% compared to a negative one.

Nature of the condition

The nature of the condition being treated is another potentially important factor. It is often believed that placebos affect only subjective symptoms like pain, anxiety or well-being. This is not quite true. Objective variables like blood tests, post-operative tissue swelling, body temperature or the healing of wounds also respond.

Yet certain conditions tend to respond better than others – pre-menstrual tension, depression, sleeplessness, migraine or other types of pain are complaints that usually respond well, but there is hardly any disease or symptom that yields no response at all.

Understanding placebo response

At present we do not fully understand all the influences on the placebo response or their possible, complex interactions. There are simply too many unknowns. One large **multi-centre study**, showed that the most important determinant of the placebo-effect was 'the centre'. In other words, even within one single trial there are remarkable variations can exist from site to site, and we cannot currently define exactly why these differences occur.

Back in the early 50s, Beecher analysed several placebo controlled trials in a paper that proved influential to the present day. He concluded that, on average, about one third of all patients responded to placebo therapy. This led to the misunderstanding that placebo effects contribute about 1/3 to the total therapeutic response. But this is not true. Beecher's figure was an **average**, but the range can span all the way from 0 to 100%

Some researchers also postulated that a certain type of personality, i.e. a 'placebo-responder' predisposes people to react to placebo. False again! Research over the last decades has failed to identify psychological traits characterising responders as opposed to non-responders. The individual who shows a reaction to placebo today may not respond tomorrow and vice versa.

It's all in the mind

A further misunderstanding claims that 'it is all in the mind'. This notion is made unlikely by a number of facts. Placebos behave pharmacologically much like drugs; they elicit dose– and time- dependent effects, and placebo reactions can cumulate just as one would expect after administering 'real' drugs. Moreover, as mentioned above, placebos also affect objective signs – anything from cholesterol levels to hair loss.

Adverse effects

Having established that placebos are potentially powerful – we might ask whether they can generate **adverse-effects**. The answer is yes! On average, some 20% of healthy volunteers and 35% of patients report adverse-effects after placebo pills; the variation is large – again probably ranging from 0% – 100%.

Many placebo-controlled drug trials show that the adverse-effects, observed in placebo-treated patients, behave in parallel with the adverse-effects of those receiving the experimental treatment. If, in one trial, a drug is tested which causes headache, the placebo group will also report headache. If, in another trial, the experimental drug causes loss of appetite, the same symptom will occur in the placebo group. We cannot be sure why this is so – possibly there is some (non-verbal?) communication between these groups. But other factors may be involved as well.

Research into placebo

After a flurry of interest in the 1950s, research into placebo became almost an exotic side-line of medical research tinted with the suspicion of quackery. Most researchers saw the placebo-effect as the 'background noise' in a clinical experiment, a nuisance that was not to be researched but accounted for through adequate study designs and controls. This attitude is presently changing. Some clinicians now remember just how beneficial placebos can be in their daily practice and aim at optimising rather than suppressing it. If a clinician doesn't elicit a powerful placebo response, they say, he/she has chosen the wrong profession. Others still have conceptual problems with this notion and fear that knowingly prescribing placebos is being dishonest and means 'cheating' the patient.

The 'ineffective yet helpful' paradox

Whenever a CAM therapy has failed to pass the test of scientific scrutiny, one often hears from its proponents that it may be 'ineffective in that sense' but it still helps a lot of people. This apparent paradox is puzzling and in many ways fascinating.

At first glance, one might detect several meanings of the 'ineffective but helpful' paradox. Most obviously it could imply that, in a clinical trial a certain therapy failed to reach a positive result for the primary outcome measure, say survival of cancer patients, but showed a positive effect in a more subtle way, for instance, **quality of life**. Thus one could claim it was ineffective for what it was tested, while it could still be helpful in other ways.

This interpretation of the 'ineffective yet helpful' paradox must, however, be rejected – not because the scenario does not exist but because it does not describe an ineffective therapy, rather it describes a poor trial. The scenario would merely refer to a trial with the wrong **primary outcome measure**. If we re-designed that study using quality of life as a **primary endpoint**, we would doubtlessly demonstrate effectiveness. 'Ineffective yet helpful' would thus not apply in this case.

Inadequate RCT

Another meaning of the 'ineffective yet helpful' paradox could refer to the inadequacy of the **randomised clinical trial** (RCT) for testing effectiveness of certain interventions, including CAM. We all know that the RCT is not perfect. It certainly can, under certain circumstances, produce **false negative results**. When this is so, the 'ineffective (as suggested by the results of a false negative RCT) yet helpful (as demonstrated by patients' experience)' notion could rightly apply. In such cases the solution would lie in defining what elements of the trail design were inappropriate and to plan a study that overcomes these problems.

Non-specific response

The most frequent use of the 'ineffective yet helpful' argument is to suggest that a therapy has no specific effect but generates a substantial non-specific (placebo) response. Thus a scientist testing it against placebo is likely to call it 'ineffective'. Nevertheless patients experience benefit from it. There could be several reasons for this discrepancy.

The most obvious is that patients benefit from a placebo effect. In everyday practice, neither the patient nor the therapist normally have reliable ways of differentiating the precise cause for clinical improvement. It could be any of:

- · a placebo effect,
- · the **natural history of the disease**,
- · **concomitant therapies**,
- · **social desirability** and, of course,
- · a **specific effect** of the therapy applied.

Generally speaking, clinicians tend to claim that it was the therapy that helped, while neglecting the other possibilities.

The power of the placebo

It would be foolish to deny the power of the placebo or to think of it as useless. But it is nevertheless important to be exact and honest about what we are dealing with and to differentiate between specific and non-specific therapeutic effects as clearly as we can.

A treatment without specific effects (i.e. one that is not superior to placebo) can be called ineffective by investigators while patients find it effective. For the patient, this may look like splitting hairs – all he or she wants is to get better. However, for medical research, and I would say for progress in general, it matters greatly.

Depending on what type of therapy was used as a 'vehicle' to 'transport' the placebo effect, different reasons come into mind. If a therapy carries significant risks, we have to ask ourselves whether the placebo response might not be 'transported' via a less risky treatment. If it is expensive, we might look for a cheaper and equally effective placebo. If it means that patients are led to believe in irrational or absurd things, we probably could find a placebo where this is less likely. Crucially, we must remember that we don't need a placebo for generating a placebo-response. Even the most efficacious treatments come with the free bonus of a placebo-effect.

Finally, there are two more issues: scientific honesty and progress. Honesty is a value in itself that, in my view, cannot be rated high enough. Progress is equally important, I think.

Significant therapeutic advances could be made if we started seriously wondering what exactly the placebo response is. If we simply are content with the view 'as long as it helps patients, all is fine', and if we don't try to define the exact causes of clinical improvement, we are unlikely to make progress. As the placebo effect is potentially powerful we should try to unpack the contents of this '**black box**'. Once we understand it better, we probably can use it better – and this would really be progress.

Evidence-Based Medicine (EBM)

The concept of **evidence-based medicine** is simple: establish and update the best evidence for all medical and therapeutic interventions through the rigorous use of accepted criteria and subsequently make sure that this knowledge is implemented in clinical practice. Simple on paper, but not quite so simple in real life!

Resistance to EBM

Having promoted evidence-based medicine for many years, I ask myself, why is there so much resistance to evidence-based medicine? In trying to answer this question I have gradually come to the conclusion that mainly five different groups of professionals hold the fort for 'non-evidence-based medicine'. They do so for dramatically different reasons.

1. The 'freedom-conscious' clinician fears that evidence-based medicine will eventually result in 'cook book medicine': diagnose Condition X, look it up in your 'cook book' and apply the optimal treatment. Clinicians would, in this scenario, be degraded to mere diagnosticians and would lose a substantial part of their liberty. This fear is real, and evidence-based medicine might, in fact, partly develop in this direction, particularly if regulators and politicians have their say.

   I do think, however, that it will also develop a new freedom – to be able to choose from a range of treatments are evidence-based, i.e. that have a high chance of helping the patient. I see no loss in throwing overboard treatments that, after rigorous testing, are demonstrably inefficient. And I see plenty of progress in developing a therapeutic tool kit of treatments that have been properly tested and thus do reliably generate more good than harm.

2. The empathic clinician may feel that evidence-based medicine is all technical and scientific, while the patient foremost needs empathy and understanding. The notion here is basically that the art and science of medicine are mutually exclusive. It is hard to deny that, this is how medicine has developed over the last few decades. This is most regrettable. But I find it difficult to agree that evidence-based medicine has caused or aggravated this development. On the contrary, I think that evidence-based medicine might, one day, enforce the value of empathy and caring by generating good evidence to show just how important these factors are.

3. The basic researchers are somewhat puzzled by evidence-based medicine, often to the extent of rejecting it. Having spent their whole professional lives in finding out how drugs and other treatments work, they suddenly find that interest in their work might be declining. True, evidence-based medicine is not directly focused on mechanisms of actions of treatments. It merely asks 'does it work?' But no one in their right mind would dream of concluding that basic research is therefore less important. On the contrary, every evidence-based medicine proponent I know agrees on the undiminished place of basic research in medicine.

4. The 'empirical' clinician is disturbed by the low value that evidence-based medicine places on all types of uncontrolled clinical data (e.g. case reports, traditional use of a therapy). True evidence-based medicine heavily relies on the results of the results of **randomised clinical trials** and **systematic reviews** or **meta-analyses** of RCTs. I think the reasons for this preference are sound. But I also know that proponents of evidence-based medicine do not disregard the essential role played by empirical data and experience. After all, empirical evidence is essential for generating hypotheses.. Once we have a hypothesis, we need to test it; and for that we need clinical trials.

5. The ignorant clinician deeply dislikes all change and so dislikes evidence-based medicine. He/she does not understand the principles of evidence-based medicine and finds it tedious to keep up with all the new information it generates. Hence such

people want nothing to do with it. They may be anti-scientific in an almost emotional way – always ready to quote myths (e.g. 'with all this science and research we have not improved the prognosis of cancer patients') and often longing for 'the good old times'. To this type of clinician, I can only say, wake up, take your blinkers off, look around you and start reading the medical literature. 'The good old times' in medicine were neither good, nor will they ever come back.

Absence of evidence is not evidence of absence

An often quoted principle holds that absence of evidence (of therapeutic benefit or risk) must not be confused with evidence of absence (of benefit or risk). The principle is undoubtedly correct and important. At first sight it also seems fairly straightforward but it has been interpreted in more than one way.

Problems start when we ask, what is 'evidence'? Some would say that personal or collective experience amounts to evidence. The above principle, however, makes little sense if anecdotes are substituted for evidence. The principle is valid only if evidence has the meaning that evidence-based medicine has given this term.

When applied to therapeutic **efficacy**, we understand the above principle to mean the following: whenever there is no compelling trial data in favour of a given therapy, this does not mean that this therapy does not work. Some might conclude from such a statement that it is still responsible to use or recommend that treatment because it might be efficacious.

Others will argue, and I tend to agree with their view, that we require more than the mere hope of efficacy – we need positive proof to issue positive recommendations. Uncertainty about efficacy foremost means one thing: we need conclusive data which defines or refutes efficacy. In other words, it should prompt us to do the research but not normally to use or recommend the therapy in question for routine healthcare.

When applied to therapeutic risk, the above-named principle is perhaps even more important: absence of evidence of risk must not be confused with evidence of absence of risk. As long as we are unsure whether Treatment X causes harm, we must not assume it to be risk-free. This looks perfectly obvious, but what are we to conclude?

Few would opt for a liberal interpretation along the following lines: as long as there is no definitive evidence of risk, it is all right to use or recommend Therapy X. We should not tolerate that patients are submitted to risks while we are uncertain about the harm this could do. The wisest conclusion from the above principle as applied to safety may therefore be the following: Therapy X has to be regarded as unsafe until positive evidence of its safety is available.

Having dissected the 'absence of evidence' principle in this way, we now see that two important principles can be derived from it.

- Firstly, any medical intervention has to be categorised as inefficacious until proven otherwise.
- Secondly, every therapy has to be considered unsafe until there is positive proof of its safety.

These are general axioms which obviously have the purpose of safeguarding the position of the patient.

It is the nature of principles that they apply across the board, i.e. for all areas of medicine. This means that the above-named principle must pertain to all therapeutic interventions. Yet one does not have to search far to find 'pockets' where they seem to be suspended: psychotherapy, surgery, physical therapy and, of course, CAM.

Rather than turning a blind eye to these exceptions, we should identify such areas of 'insufficient evidence' and work towards filling the existing gaps in our knowledge – and this would be not because we aim to comply with a theoretical principle or to fulfil the needs of those working in academic 'ivory towers', it would be because we all want to act in the best interests of our patients.

Publish or Perish

Maybe I am hopelessly over-optimistic, but I expect that, having read this book, you now understand enough about research methodology to start to read research articles in your field. Over time, this would gradually increase your comprehension and interest in healthcare and matters of research.

As this happens, one day, you might even feel tempted to write and publish an article in a medical journal yourself. I would certainly encourage you to try. During the last 30 years, I have published more papers than I care to remember. Essentially this means that I have committed all the mistakes one can possibly make. So perhaps I truly am in a good position to offer a few tips about how to avoid them.

Read research articles

The most important thing is probably to read medical articles regularly. If nothing else, this keeps you informed and teaches you how medical papers are written. My suggestion is that, each week you read for 2 to 3 hours in and around your field of interest.

Once you have a vague idea for an article, let it settle and inform yourself on what others have published on the same or similar subjects. There are, of course, different types of articles.

- Editorials are often invited by the editors of journals.
- Comments or opinion pieces are exactly what they say they are. They need to be thought-provoking and succinct.

- Letters are short communications on articles that a journal has previously published; they thrive on views that the original authors may have omitted.
- Reviews require sound knowledge of the subject and are best conceived as **systematic reviews**.
- Original research papers are the most prestigious of the lot. They obviously require that you have conducted original research.
- **Case reports** or **case series** may be a much more realistic option for busy clinicians. These should focus on truly remarkable cases and must provide a complete account of what these cases were about.

There are virtually thousands of medical journals including CAM journals, specialist journals for nurses, physiotherapists etc.

Select the appropriate article

If you want to submit an article for publication, make sure that you choose the right one. Clearly it must be in the subject area of your paper, and your article must fit the requirements of your journal of choice. So familiarise yourself with the options, chose carefully, and pitch your article correctly for that journal.

Structure

Before you start writing, jot down a 'line of thought' that you want to follow. In the case of original research papers this structure is dictated by convention (see page 31). But, for other types of communications, you have much more freedom. Your paper will only be gripping if you follow a clear sequence of thought. There is nothing more tiring than reading an article that has no structure, is full of repetitions and omissions and seems to go everywhere and nowhere. This is to be avoided at all costs.

Draft and renew

Once you have a structure, draft the text. Then put it aside for 2-3 days. This enables you to gain some distance and see it with new eyes. Subsequently revise your draft and repeat this cycle until you find that there is nothing you want to change. My own articles often go through more than 10 revisions – so don't be impatient. **Critical assessment** can be difficult at the best of times, but when it relates to your own work, it is very hard.

Now you have a well-written article. At this stage it might be a good idea to show it to someone else and invite constructive criticism. In my experience, this step often proves invaluable. Of course, the downside is that you may have to start another cycle of revision if your friend's comments recommend it.

Submission

Finally you have the finished product which you can submit to the journal of your choice. Compose a good covering letter to go with it. This might explain why you feel this article is important at this particular moment. The editor will most likely send your article to 2 or 3 peer reviewers. They will provide a written critique of your work which you should take most seriously. In other words, another cycle of revisions may ensue. In the end, you will have something you can be proud of.

Publishing is a tough business. Be under no illusions that it might be all plain-sailing. The process is time and energy consuming and often infuriating. But, with a bit of luck, it comes to the right conclusion: a paper with your name on it. This will give you satisfaction like little else in life. It can also further your career. But, most importantly, it teaches you a lot and you will be a better practitioner for it.

Footnote

There are, of course, numerous courses on how to get published. The Royal Society of Medicine, for instance, offers one (**www.rsm.ac.uk/yf/yfmeet.htm**)

CHAPTER 8 **APPENDICES**

Appendix 1

Relevant websites

Association of Medical Research Charities – **www.amrc.org.uk**

Clinical Trials Unit (MRC) – **www.ctu.mrc.ac.uk/TrialInfo.asp**

INVOLVE – **http://invo.org.uk**

The James Lind Library – **www.jameslindlibrary.org**

Medical Research Council – **www.mrc.ac.uk**

National Institutes for Health Research – **www.nihr.ac.uk**

National Library for Health (NHS) – **www.library.nhs.uk/trials**

Pharmaceutical Industry Clinical Trials database – **www.cmrinteract.com/clintrial**

UK Clinical Research Collaboration – **www.ukcrc.org**

UK Clinical Research Network – **www.ukcrn.org.uk**.

The US National Institutes of Health Clinical Trials – **www.clinicaltrials.gov**

Appendix 2

Ten recent important CAM research reports

- Mazieres B, Hucher M, Zaim M, Garnero P. Effect of chondroitin sulfate in symptomatic knee osteoarthritis: A multicenter, randomized, double blind, placebo-controlled study. Ann Rheum Deis 2007; doi: 10.1136/ard.2006.059899

- Jacobs J, Fernandez EA, Merizalde B, Avila-Montes GA, Crothers D. The use of homeopathic combination remedy for dengue fever symptoms: a pilot RCT in Honduras. Homeopathy 2007; 96: 22-26

- Robertson A, Suryanarayanan R, Banerjee A. Homeopathic Arnica Montana for posttonsillectomy analgesia: a randomized placebo control. Homeopathy. 2007; 96: 17-21

- Perlman AI, Sabina A, Williams AL, Njike VY, Katz DL. Massage therapy for osteoarthritis of the knee: a randomized controlled trial. Arch Intern Med 2006; 166: 2533-2538

- Zepelin HH, Meden H, Kostev K, Schröder-Bernhardt D, Stammwitz U, Becher H. Isopropanolic black cohosh extract and recurrence-free survival after breast cancer. Int J Clin Pharmacol Ther 2007; 45: 143-154

- Bjelakovic G, Nikolova D, Gluud LL, Simonetti RG, Gludd C. Mortality in randomized trials of antioxidant supplements for primary and secondary prevention. JAMA 2007; 297: 842-857

- Eisenberg DM, Post DE, Davis RB, Connelly MT, Legedza AT, Hrbek AL, Prosser LA, Buring JE, Inui TS, Cherkin DC. Addition of choice of complementary therapies to usual care for acute low back pain: a randomized controlled trial.

- Mautrie N, Campbell AM, Whyte F, McConnachie A, Emslie C, Lee R, Kearny N, Walker A, Ritchie D. Benefits of supervised groups exercise programmge for women being treated for early stage breast cancer: pragmatic randomized controlled trial. Br Med J 2007; 334: 517-523

- Mehling WE, Jacobs B, Acree M, Wilson L, Bostrom A, West J, Acquah J, Burns B, Chapman J, Hecht FM. Symptom management with massage and acupuncture in postoperative cancer patients: a randomized controlled trial. J Pain symptom Manage 2007; 33: 258-266

- Wilkinson SM, Love SB, Westcombe AM, Gambles MA, Burgess CC, Cargill A, Young T, Maher J, Ramirez AJ. Effectiveness of aromatherapy massage in the management of anxiety and depression in patients with cancer: a multicenter randomized controlled trial. J Clin Oncol 2007; 25: 532-539

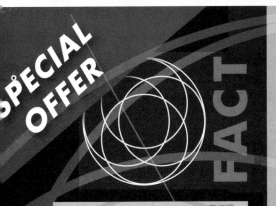

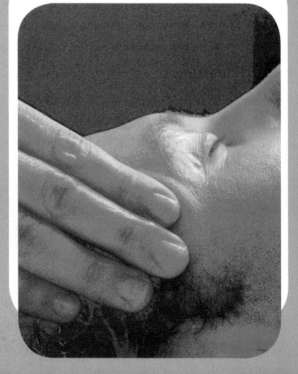
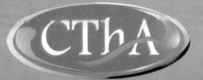